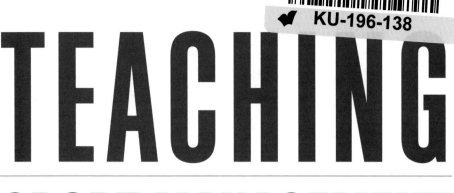

TEACHING
SPORT MANAGEMENT

A PRACTICAL GUIDE

DINA GENTILE, EdD
Professor, Sport Management
Endicott College

JONES AND BARTLETT PUBLISHERS
Sudbury, Massachusetts
BOSTON   TORONTO   LONDON   SINGAPORE

World Headquarters

Jones and Bartlett Publishers
40 Tall Pine Drive
Sudbury, MA 01776
978-443-5000
info@jbpub.com
www.jbpub.com

Jones and Bartlett Publishers
Canada
6339 Ormindale Way
Mississauga, Ontario L5V 1J2
Canada

Jones and Bartlett Publishers
International
Barb House, Barb Mews
London W6 7PA
United Kingdom

Jones and Bartlett's books and products are available through most bookstores and
online booksellers. To contact Jones and Bartlett Publishers directly, call 800-832-0034,
fax 978-443-8000, or visit our website www.jbpub.com.

Substantial discounts on bulk quantities of Jones and Bartlett's publications are available to
corporations, professional associations, and other qualified organizations. For details and specific
discount information, contact the special sales department at Jones and Bartlett via the above
contact information or send an email to specialsales@jbpub.com.

Production Credits
Acquisitions Editor: Shoshanna Goldberg
Senior Associate Editor: Amy L. Bloom
Editorial Assistant: Kyle Hoover
Production Manager: Julie Champagne Bolduc
Production Assistant: Jessica Steele Newfell
Associate Marketing Manager: Jody Sullivan
V.P., Manufacturing and Inventory Control: Therese Connell
Composition: International Typesetting and Composition
Cover Design: Kristin E. Parker
Assistant Photo Researcher: Bridget Kane
Cover Image: © Jason Stitt/ShutterStock, Inc.
Printing and Binding: Malloy, Inc.
Cover Printing: Malloy, Inc.

Library of Congress Cataloging-in-Publication Data
Gentile, Dina.
  Teaching sport management : a practical guide / Dina Gentile.
    p. cm.
  Includes bibliographical references and index.
  ISBN 978-0-7637-6672-6 (pbk. : alk. paper)
  1. Sports administration—Study and teaching. 2. Sports—Management—Study and teaching.
I. Title.
  GV713.G46 2010
  796.06'9—dc22
                                                                        2009015394
6048
Printed in the United States of America
13 12 11 10 09   10 9 8 7 6 5 4 3 2 1

To Laine and Quinn:
For your daily inspiration and for teaching me how
to smile, laugh, and love. You are my two precious gifts.
Forever, Your MaDi

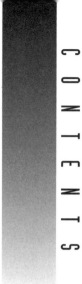

CONTENTS

PREFACE xiii

ACKNOWLEDGMENTS xix

CHAPTER 1
Teaching Sport Management 1

Sport Management Today 2
- What Is Sport Management? 2
- Evolution of Sport Management Programs of Study 3
- Accreditation and Sport Management 4

Learning Goals 9
- Building on Prior Knowledge 10
- Course Activities: Issues of Consistency and Duplication 11
- Assessment Activities 11
- Engaging Students 14

Integrating Technology Tools 20
- Guide to Incorporating Technology Into the Sport Management Curriculum 20
- New Territory: Web-Enhanced Courses 21

Questions to Consider 23

CHAPTER 2
Teaching Activities: Foundation of Sport Management 25

Sport Leadership 26
- Activity I: Sport Management Interest Group Formation 26
- Activity II: Effective Management and Leadership 27

█ Activity III: Successful Managers   28

█ Activity IV: Current Leaders in the Sport
Management Industry   28

█ Activity V: Campus Leaders in Sport and Athletics   29

Internships and Careers   29

█ Activity I: Internship Discovery   29

█ Activity II: Internship Poster Presentation or
Virtual Poster Presentation   31

█ Activity III: Portfolio Reflection—Internship Discovery   32

Strategic Planning   34

█ Activity I: Sport Business Research   34

Resume Writing   37

█ Activity I: Who Am I?   37

█ Activity II: Feedback   37

█ Activity III: Revisions   37

█ Activity IV: Interview Questions   37

█ Activity V: The Interview   38

Questions to Consider   38

CHAPTER 3
Teaching Activities: Sport Organization
Management and Administration   39

Sport Organization Management and
Administration   40

█ Activity I: Formation of Institution   40

█ Activity II: Conference Affiliation   40

█ Activity III: Mission Statement Development   41

█ Activity IV: Schedule Development   42

█ Activity V: Travel Needs   49

█ Activity VI: Contract Signing   50

█ Activity VII: Contest Management   51

█ Activity VIII: Playing the Games   53

█ Activity IX: State of Athletics   54

█ Activity X: Off-Season Tournament Development   54

█ Activity XI: Hiring Plan   55

█ Activity XII: Written Institutional Policies and Procedures   55

█ Activity XIII: Website Development   58

█ Activity XIV: Professional Presentation   58

Questions to Consider   59

CHAPTER 4
Teaching Activities: Financial Management   **60**

Organization of Lecture and Class Discourse   61

▐ Class Discussion   62

▐ Activity I: Interview With a Financial
Manager in Sports   62

▐ Activity II: Budget Creation and Decision-Making
Simulation   64

▐ Activity III: Budget Creation and Analysis   65

▐ Activity IV: Stock Market Awareness   66

▐ Activity V: Stock Ownership   67

▐ Activity VI: Financial Management Group Work   70

▐ Activity VII: Business Plan Creation and Analysis   71

Advanced Topics in Sport Management   72

▐ Activity I: Examining Leagues   72

▐ Activity II: League Think   73

▐ Activity III: Comparison of National Versus
International Leagues   73

Questions to Consider   74

CHAPTER 5
Teaching Activities: Sport Marketing and
Sport Sponsorship   **75**

Sport Marketing Sectors of Sport Management   76

▐ Activity I: Sport Product or Service Invention   78

▐ Activity II: Sport Sponsorship Event Creation From
Start to Finish   86

▐ Activity III: Sport Promotion Success or Failure   87

▐ Activity IV: Sport Personalities and Marketing   87

▐ Activity V: Impact of Sport Products on the
Industry   88

▐ Activity VI: Change the School Mascot   88

▐ Activity VII: Adopt a Team   89

▐ Activity VIII: Advertisements and Sport:
An Interactive Project   89

▐ Activity IX: Charitable Causes and Sport   91

▐ Activity X: Creation of a New Intramural League   91

▐ Activity XI: Online Discussion Board Technology   91

▐ Activity XII: Student Summary and Thoughts   91

▌ Activity XIII: Careers in Sport Marketing   92

▌ Activity XIV: Branding and Slogan Competition   93

▌ Activity XV: Create a Publicity Campaign   93

▌ Activity XVI: Professional Athletes and
  Endorsements   93

Questions to Consider   94

CHAPTER 6
International Perspective on Sport
Management   95

Case Study Analysis   96

▌ Activity I: Journal Presentation–Global
  Landscape Q & A   97

▌ Activity II: International Marketplace   97

▌ Activity III: Globalization of Professional Sport   99

▌ Activity IV: Debates   100

Questions to Consider   101

CHAPTER 7
Legal Aspects of Sport   102

Legal Aspects   103

▌ Activity I: Competency Statements   103

▌ Activity II: Sport Law Professional Portfolio   103

▌ Activity III: Topics of Study in the Legal Domain   104

▌ Activity IV: Legal Debates   104

▌ Activity V: Legal Case Study Debates   104

▌ Activity VI: Legal Brief   105

▌ Activity VII: Research in Sport Law   105

▌ Activity VIII: Sport Governing Bodies   106

▌ Activity IX: Sport Governance Research   106

Questions to Consider   107

CHAPTER 8
Teaching With Technology   108

Technology and Sport Management   109

Electronic Portfolio Implementation   111

▌ Getting Started: From a Professor's Perspective   112

▌ Getting Started: From a Student's Perspective   113

▌ Student Needs   113

▌ Troubleshooting   113

▌ e-Portfolio: Course Material   114
▌ Starting the e-Portfolio Process   114
▌ Sample Contents for e-Portfolios: Introductory
  Sport Management Course   114
▌ e-Portfolio Presentation   116
Learner-Centered Teaching   119
Tools of the Industry   119
Questions to Consider   120

CHAPTER 9
Outcomes Assessment   121
Assessment Defined   122
Program Goals and Mission   122
Outcomes for the Sport Management Major   124
Student Learning Outcomes   124
Assessment Tools for Sport Management   126
Student Evaluations and Course Objectives:
  Informal Process of Evaluation   128
Sport Management Faculty United   129
Questions to Consider   131

CHAPTER 10
Putting It All Together   132
Course Syllabus: Where to Start?   133
Course Content   134
Online Course Development   136
▌ Course Introduction   136
▌ Faculty Welcome Message   136
▌ Course Objectives   137
▌ Topical Outline   137
▌ Rubric for Discussion Forum Participation   137
▌ Due Dates and Due Times   137
Organizing Course Materials   137
Advising Responsibilities   138
▌ Registration Process   138
▌ Progress Reports   138
Mentoring Students   139
▌ Office Hours   139
▌ E-Mail Correspondence   139

Value Added: Speaker Series   139

▌ Background Information on Guest Speaker   139

▌ Student Engagement During Guest Speaker Presentation   140

▌ Speaker Series Review   140

Exit Interviews   140

Sport Management Today and Beyond   141

INDEX   142

PHOTO CREDITS   147

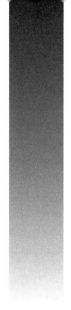

Preface

Teaching sport management has never been more exciting and challenging. Now, a desk-side companion text exists to provide sport management educators with the tips and tools necessary to teach the most common course offerings within sport management education: *Teaching Sport Management: A Practical Guide.* Updated teaching techniques can serve as a primer for sport management educators who are hungry for innovative teaching activities and ideas to incorporate technology into the curriculum. Essential content areas for the effective delivery of sport management programs include navigating the accreditation process, course and program assessment, electronic portfolio integration, technology integration, course content guidelines, syllabus development, online and hybrid course preparation, and teaching tools and techniques. Guidelines and tips are shared that outline practical implementation ideas for the delivery of high-level sport management education. The primary intent and goal of *Teaching Sport Management: A Practical Guide* is to share information and foster creativity in sport management curricula. Sport management educators will find tools and concepts that can be easily incorporated into their classrooms.

Sport Management Today

Sport management, as an academic major, has experienced a remarkable growth in enrollment and interest over the last 30 years. From an academic standpoint, sport management educators—now more than ever—are preparing sport management students for a dynamic industry filled with change, problems, opportunities, and challenges. From an economic standpoint, the value of educated sport professionals has increased in importance since the inception of the first sport management program in the 1960s. Today, sport organizations and businesses are seeking to hire qualified individuals who possess the skills of business executives along with the keen awareness of sport as a unique product and the understanding of sport fans as a profitable consumer group.

The responsibility of faculty members and academic administrators to deliver quality sport management education has never been so important. The academic major of sport management is heading into a new era of program accreditation. As the shift from program approval through the National Association of Sport and Physical Education–North American Society for Sport Management (NASPE–NASSM) changes to an accreditation process governed by the Commission on Sport Management Accreditation (COSMA), it is timely for sport management educators to analyze the strengths and weaknesses of our academic programs of study. Now is the best time for the focus to be centered on teaching strategies, assessment, and learner engagement. These essential components of sport management education must become or continue to be primary areas of concentration and improvement for sport management educators.

The proverbial sport management "bar" has been raised, and it is incumbent that sport management educators determine the standards that are essential in their courses and programs. It is timely for faculty members and deans to work in tandem to ensure the proper and effective delivery of their sport management education to students. In order to produce quality programs of study, a link between faculty members and academic administrators needs to be strengthened. Open discussions and information sharing by both parties serve to connect the responsibilities and roles of all "players" within sport management education. This text can serve as the link to showcase the opportunities for growth in sport management education while providing unique and practical ideas of teaching methodology to enhance the "in and out of classroom experiences" for all sport management students.

The sport management curriculum has been evolving over the last decade. The sheer volume of sport management programs throughout the United States, Europe, Australia, and New Zealand demonstrates the strength and broad appeal of this type of major. We have moved from program approval (where institutions would submit documents of information to a governing body) to a more thorough and complete evaluation of the types of academic degrees we are offering and granting to students. NASPE–NASSM has made strides to create a uniform system of program approval, which will now be governed by COSMA. Sport management is following in the footsteps of its cousins, Physical Education and Athletic Training. The move from a paper trail of proof in the former model of approval to an intensive examination of the program of study including outcome assessment is one of the reasons *Teaching Sport Management: A Practical Guide* was written.

Sport management faculty members and academic deans should rethink or re-create the methodology of determining student growth and learning within the sport management curriculum. Many questions arise when we think about what a sport management program should look like: what courses should be included, what course content is appropriate, what is the ideal sequence of course offerings, and who is qualified to teach these courses? Ideally, our students should be able to effectively lead, manage, direct, and develop sport management organizations in all of the various sectors of the industry. We, of course, want our students to be well-rounded and liberally educated so that they can critically attack the issues at hand and make ethical decisions when confronted with managerial dilemmas. How do we start to re-invent a curriculum that has been part of our institution for so many years? Or better yet, do we need to re-invent the curriculum? *Teaching Sport Management: A Practical Guide* sheds light on how to make your sport management program today's sport management program. From an optimistic perspective, COSMA gives institutions the start it needs to formalize the sport management curriculum; add course content that teaches students the important aspects of the major; and provide integrity to sport management programs, which have often been categorized and unfairly labeled as "sports major." Some of us may still debate where we should appropriately house our program. The question of sport management as a stand-alone major or embedded within schools of business has been an ongoing debate since sport management's inception and ultimate popularity on college campuses. An accrediting body and all of the ins and outs that come with such an approval process will surely add a level of prestige to institutions seeking this external accreditation and the ultimate stamp of approval from the sport management governing body.

As we move into a new era of accreditation, it is important for sport management educators to understand the strides of sport management over the last three decades. NASPE–NASSM has been instrumental in examining common content areas and faculty member credentials in sport management programs at both the graduate and undergraduate levels.

Technology and Sport Management

The rapid growth and use of information technology by the general public has led to an explosion of computer software applications and usage both at home and in the workplace. Sport management faculty members will need to be competent in the use and delivery of common technology to provide enriching, dynamic courses to students who rely on their guidance and expertise to prepare them for careers in the sport business industry. As technology continues to stretch from home use to business use and beyond, sport management faculty members must start to rethink and embrace methods for teaching with technology. The information presented in this text is timely, in that more and more faculty members are starting to teach courses that use technology, courses that are hybrid in nature (sessions in class and sessions in cyber space), and courses that are delivered completely online. *Teaching Sport Management: A Practical Guide* recognizes that technology has changed the way we communicate in society as a whole, and it strongly emphasizes that we need to share this timely information with sport management educators in order to effectively integrate technology into the classroom. On the one hand, this information will allow professors to enhance teaching strategies, and, on the other hand, our sport management students will be effectively prepared for future opportunities and will be better educated through contemporary and forward-thinking learning activities embedded into course lessons and assignments.

In the end, our sport management students will be able to use the technology/computer experience gained throughout the curriculum as an advantage as they market themselves for internship or career positions in the field. Within the proceeding chapters, sport management educators will find the information can be used for the traditional classroom setting and also adapted for those who use hybrid or fully online courses. The concepts, research, and ideas detailed in this text allow sport management educators to effectively educate their students and to incorporate practical models for applying and combining computer technology with instructional methods and resources through in-class activities and out-of-class assignments.

Organization of the Book

At the onset, *Teaching Sport Management: A Practical Guide* provides an overview of the sport management discipline. The subsequent chapters provide an overview of concepts and ideas to enhance student learning within the most common types of sport management courses. In addition, the *Teaching Tip* sections embedded in each chapter provide readers with specific teaching and instructional techniques that can be applied to a wide array of sport management specific courses. The text uses a number of common courses within the sport management program of study to provide tips, tools, and guides for teaching the most appropriate and significant content. The text also addresses tools that can be utilized in traditional classroom settings, hybrid courses, and fully online courses along with an exploration of future trends in the discipline of sport management, from course content and instructional innovations to improvements in technological tools. At the end of each chapter, readers can reflect and respond to the *Questions to Consider* section.

The unique aspect of this text is that no other publication exists to supplement the sport management educators' teaching toolbox covering multiple courses within the sport management curriculum. *Teaching Sport Management: A Practical Guide* is a tremendous resource for first-time instructors and established sport management faculty members. For the first time a resource exists to specifically assist sport management educators in becoming more sensitive to their teaching effectiveness and, more importantly, to ensure student learning and acquisition of knowledge.

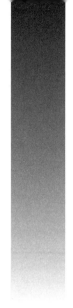

Acknowledgments

This book was written from my passion to teach and to create unique learning environments for my students. Thanks to all of my sport management students for inspiring me to deliver innovative and challenging course activities to spark your interest in the field. Your passion to learn and your trust in completing these learning activities have motivated me to write this book.

Special thanks to my family for supporting me in this process and allowing me the time to think and to write.

Thanks and appreciation to the reviewers of this text for providing detailed comments on the content and delivery of the material: Dr. Susan E. Langlois, Springfield College, and Dr. Chrystal D. Porter, Endicott College.

Finally, thanks to the Jones and Bartlett family, for making the journey of putting this material together into a comprehensive text smooth and enjoyable. Special thanks to Amy Bloom, Jess Newfell, and Kyle Hoover, who have been terrific guides in this endeavor.

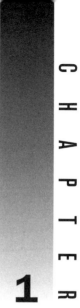

Teaching Sport Management

Sport management as an academic discipline is without a doubt experiencing tremendous growth. As these programs of study flourish, courses and course content need to reflect the dynamic and innovative industry that is sport business. All sport management programs of study, as we move into a new era of accreditation, should take the time to review, create, and reflect on their courses and the effectiveness of the embedded course content along with evaluating the teaching and learning that occurs throughout a student's academic career.

In this chapter we explore the following components:
- Sport management defined and reviewed
- Challenges and opportunities in accreditation
- Teaching effectiveness in sport management
- Teaching with technology

Sport Management Today

What Is Sport Management?

If I had a nickel for every person who has asked me this question, I would be rich! Most of us who teach in sport management have answered this question a multitude of times and each time we do it with passion and with a smile on our face. Often times, prospective students and families just assume our major is just about sports! Subsequently, it is often assumed that because a student has played a sport for a number of years that sport knowledge transfers into sport management knowledge. The wonderful aspect of teaching first-year students is that you have a chance to enlighten them on sport management and the variety of opportunities within the sport business industry. Many students are often unaware of the academic discipline simply because they have not been exposed to the vast nature and wide array of career and professional opportunities within the sport business industry. Students are often attracted to the sport management major from their past experiences as an athlete or from their passion for sport.

Regardless of the motivation for selecting sport management as a major area of focus, the sport management educator's role is to expose students to the major and to reveal the impact of sport management on society today both at the national and international levels. The business of sport has become more and more focused on management skills, economic decision making, budgeting, and leadership of small and large sport entities.

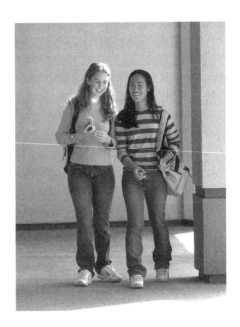

Students who apply to major in the discipline of sport management almost need to be reprogrammed in their thinking about what sport management entails and the career opportunities that are presented to them.

Evolution of Sport Management Programs of Study

While searching for the definition of sport management one may discover a slew of common definitions. Pitts and Stotlar (2002) referred to sport management as "all people, activities, businesses, and organizations involved in producing facilitating, promoting, or organizing any product that is sport, fitness, and recreation related" (p. 4). The umbrella that is sport management covers a vast variety of career paths for our students. Davis (1994) used a practical and accurate depiction of the industry by revealing that "sport managers are the wonderful glue that binds successful sport organizations, sport events, athletes, health clubs, and virtually every sport industry-related business" (p. 5). Sport management can very well be considered an umbrella industry where the focus centers on sport as a product and the ribs of the parasol are the vast opportunities that exist within the sport industry. The flexible nature of sport management adds to its broad appeal as this academic major attracts a large number of prospective college students.

Over 200 programs are listed by the North American Society for Sport Management (NASSM). However, only a relatively small percentage of those member institutions have actually received program approval status from the Sport Management Program Review Council (SMPRC). Laird (2005) revealed a surprising statistic that approximately 75% of member institutions were not identified as approved programs. With low numbers of institutions seeking program approval from the governing association, it begs the question: How many member institutions

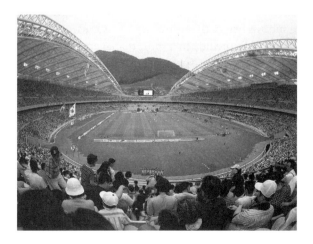

will shy away from the newly created and established accreditation process? The switch to prepare for the accreditation process and all it entails presents challenges for many sport management institutions as we move forward.

Sport management as a discipline will be closely examined by academicians as we progress into new standards and principles associated with accreditation. To gain accreditation status institutions must take an even closer look at the courses offered, course content, projects, textbooks and readings, and assessment tools, along with critical mass and credentials of sport management faculty members. Although many may be apprehensive about the accreditation journey, the idea that sport management programs across the nation are thoroughly examined and held to consistent standards adds credibility to our academic discipline and provides an even playing field across institutions, because all sport management programs will be susceptible to the same requirements. Moreover, visiting accreditation teams can also assist programs in providing recommendations to strengthen course offerings and assessment, reinforce the strengths of the program, and provide guidance and make suggestions for areas of need and improvement.

Since the first reported graduate degree in 1966 at Ohio University (Parkhouse & Pitts, 2001) to 1989 when the National Association for Sport and Physical Education (NASPE)-NASSM Joint Committee established the approval process for programs (NASPE-NASSM, 2000) to 2007 when the Commission on Sport Management Accreditation (COSMA) manual was first published online (NASPE-NASSM, 2007), sport management has and will continue to change and adapt to satisfy industry and academic standards. In July 2008, COSMA revised its materials and manuals online to assist institutions aiming for accreditation (COSMA, 2008).

Accreditation and Sport Management

Accreditation and sport management have been a topic of discussion for many academicians before the formation of COSMA. Which courses and the type of content to include in a sport management program have been argued and debated among sport management educators over the last decades. Interestingly, Pitts (2001) identified five essential elements that should be included within an academic field of study:

1. A body of knowledge and literature as it relates to theory and practice
2. Three types of professionals (educators, researchers, and practitioners)
3. Professional organizations
4. Professional preparation
5. Credibility

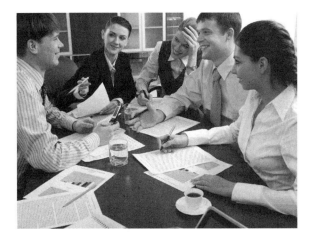

To add to that list, one of the greatest challenges for COSMA will be to communicate the standards and the process of accreditation to member institutions; Laird (2005) discovered that 21% of surveyed sport management academicians were not familiar with program approval for sport management under the NASPE-NASSM structure.

To demonstrate that accreditation has been circling sport management education for over a decade we can look to the work of Fielding, Pitts, and Miller (1991), who examined sport management educators in the area of accreditation and assessment. In one part of the study the researchers asked academicians in sport management whether they were in favor of accreditation. Over 15 years ago respondents indicated 32% were in favor of accreditation, 25% were not in favor nor opposed, and 43% opposed accreditation (Fielding et al., 1991).

A number of years have passed, and with that perhaps the thinking of the benefits of accreditation has changed as well. Sport management programs can decide whether to seek accreditation or not. Unlike academic programs of education, athletic training, and nursing, sport management graduates do not need to be licensed to practice their craft. Therefore the external pressure to seek accreditation does not currently exist for sport management programs. Students do not need to pass a standardized or industry-wide examination to demonstrate their mastery of competencies and acquisition of core knowledge. As with other licensure programs in higher education, accreditation currently is not mandated for colleges and universities that offer sport management as a degree program.

Although accreditation does assist in providing consistency in the core courses we offer in sport management, Fielding et al. (1991) also pointed out that with accreditation comes some disadvantages: loss of credibility, elitism, implementation costs, and program costs. Over the next few years it will be interesting to note and evaluate the progress institutions are making on the accreditation front.

Commission on Sport Management Accreditation

COSMA originally published a manual in 2007 to guide institutions on their quest to attain accreditation. An updated manual was posted on the COSMA website in July 2008 (COSMA, 2008). The ideal of COSMA is that sport management programs should strive for excellence in their delivery of sport management education. Defining excellence may be an obstacle for many in academia. What does it mean to be an excellent sport management program? The efforts of COSMA are certainly appreciated as we move forward and upward as an academic major. The standardized protocol within sport management adds value and creates consistency in sport management programs. COSMA also encourages academic programs to maintain their uniqueness and a sense of their own created identity. Clearly, sport management faculty members play an integral role in creating "excellent" classroom environments for students. Faculty members need to become partners in the system-wide approach to accreditation for sport management programs. The accreditation process should serve to clarify the task and mission of the sport management program and to provide yet another assessment tool for faculty members within the discipline. All involved in the accreditation process should welcome the stages of development as it keeps the program current and dynamic. More importantly, sport management educators and administrators can receive external feedback on a program they may have been working with for years and even decades to avoid any staleness that may naturally develop.

The major focus for both sport management academic administrators and faculty members should be centered on the curriculum along with outcomes derived from those courses that comprise the sport management program. COSMA does illuminate the definition of excellence:

> Excellence in sport management education requires that the design of each program offered by the academic unit/sport management program be consistent with current, acceptable practices and the expectations of professionals in the academic and sport management communities. (COSMA, 2008, p. 9)

At the heart of the accreditation documentation and process are the identified common professional components (CPC). In essence, the CPC (**Table 1.1**) provide sport management educators with a guide for the type of content that must be addressed in courses and/or throughout the 4-year program of study. For faculty members whose primary responsibility and

Table 1.1 COSMA: Common Professional Components

- Social, psychological, and international foundations of sport management
- Sport management principles
- Sport leadership
- Sport operations management/event and venue management
- Sport governance
- Ethics in sport management
- Sport marketing
- Finance/accounting/economics
- Principles of sport finance
- Accounting
- Economics of sport
- Legal aspects of sport
- Integrative experience, such as:
  - Strategic management/policy
  - Internship
  - Capstone experience

Source: Commission on Sport Management Accreditation (COSMA). (2008). Accreditation Principles and Self Study Preparation. Available at: http://iweb.aahperd.org/naspe/cosma/pdf_files/accrPrinciples.pdf. Accessed April 2, 2009.

role in the process is to be sure students learn and grow through a wide array of assessment and evaluation techniques, these standards are important to explore and investigate. Throughout the revision and creation of course syllabi, sport management educators and administrators should take the time to review the specific CPC that are incorporated into course objectives and ultimately in course outcomes and assessment. The COSMA-derived CPC are extremely similar in detail to the prevision course content requirements created by NASPE-NASSM program approval guidelines. From this perspective, it is clear the standards of sport management parallel those of SMPRC. The critical distinction is in the process in which institutions demonstrate that these components are being adequately covered and addressed in courses and that students are demonstrating growth and learning through the acquisition of knowledge gained through sport management designated courses and course topics.

Now that the common components of the profession of sport management are published and available, sport management educators must move to identify the courses in which these components rest, coupled with identifying how to evaluate these components. At a glance when looking at sport management programs, currently NASSM lists designated institutions that offer a degree in sport management from the United States, Canada, Europe, Australia, New Zealand, India, and Africa. Many predict the number of sport management programs will continue to grow with the popularity and recognition of the major through accreditation. Currently, institutions are experiencing dramatic increases in enrollment with a sport management major offering.

While reviewing curriculum offerings, the CPC in many cases and at many institutions are in fact the actual name of a course or the course title includes many of the COSMA stated terms. The COSMA document clarifies that colleges and universities do not need one singular course to cover each of these areas. Some courses naturally cover multiple components, whereas others touch on a single concept. The importance of the process of accreditation is that institutions demonstrate that these designated areas of outcomes are central to the delivery of the programs of study.

To more effectively explain the ability for institutions to reach "excellence" in their sport management program, COSMA clarifies the difference between standards and principles:

> Standards provide arbitrary cut-off points, where the standard is either met or not: while principles assess progress toward excellence, allow for a continuum of accomplishment, and encourage continuous improvement. (COSMA, 2008, p. 1)

Following that definition, if sport management educators and academic administrators focus on principles, as program stakeholders, we are capable of using our creativity and our experience teaching and engaging students to reach the prescribed principles. The broader look at the achievement of sport management excellence allows all types of institutions, large or small, to demonstrate the alignment with the approved sport management principles.

From an economic and enrollment perspective, each institution wants to have a niche in the market for sport management students. Variations do exist among sport management degree offerings however, many courses in these programs are similar in fashion. One can easily navigate the Internet to find the listing of course offerings and requirements for both graduate and undergraduate sport management programs of study. To provide organization and flow to the book, the most common courses and course topics found in sport management programs are addressed. The names and time in program of delivery of the reviewed courses and course activities vary from institution to institution. Many sport management programs share common themes, texts, and readings, which is expected of a program of study that has an accrediting or approval governing body. COSMA will, at a minimum, provide a level of consistency in the look and the content of sport management programs. Often, when institutions are seeking external approval, the curriculum becomes a prescription of courses that students must complete. Sport management programs today have the flexibility to offer courses unique to the program of student. Sport management programs should not lose the creativity in course offerings and genuineness of courses they current offer to just meet the COSMA standards. The "Outcomes Assessment Principle" designated by COSMA recognizes that all institutions find a way to deliver their own program of study.

Learning Goals

COSMA requires institutions to demonstrate that students are acquiring a knowledge base from the sport management program of study. Assessing learning goals is critical in the accreditation stage for sport management educators. As faculty members set out to teach their courses, they must have a keen awareness of what specific learning outcomes students should achieve.

As the course syllabus is developed, sport management educators can focus on identifying and clarifying the list of course objectives provided to students. The central focus of the syllabus is to present the pedagogical goals and objectives for the course. Student achievement and performances are measured using the stated course objectives. Course objectives are connected to outcomes assessment, in that sport management educators will use the objectives to measure to what extent students have met or achieved the objectives. What is the purpose of course objectives? Simply stated, course objectives are what students should learn from the content of the course. Moreover, these stated objectives become for many educators the direction of and for their teaching. There is a direct relationship between teaching goals and the written and established course objectives. Through the established course objectives, sport management educators build lectures, projects, and assignments. At the start and throughout the semester faculty members can refer back to the learning/course objectives to determine if student progress is being made toward achieving the stated objectives.

It is important to note the distinction between course objectives and the course outline. The course outline lists the content areas that will be explored and covered throughout the semester or term. Course objectives are clearly stated aims and goals of what will be taught throughout the semester or term. Sport management educators and administrators must spend time constantly reviewing the course objectives so that all stated aims are somehow being addressed through the semester and throughout the course content.

Teaching Tip

Before an exam students can be directed to review course objectives. To aid in the study process, students can try to write a response to each of the applicable course objectives. Students, through this activity, can get a sense of the importance of the listed course objectives. Students will also be able to apply their knowledge when creating a written response to the course aims.

Teaching Tip

When sport management faculty members and administrators develop rubrics for course activities and assignments, the easiest place to start is with what we expect our students to accomplish within the course, typically outlined in our course objectives section.

Sport management programs should take into account how often course objectives are updated and who has control over the process. At most institutions the course objectives have been approved by an academic assembly or governing body. Objectives typically should not be arbitrarily changed without a stamp of approval from the academic department. Again, for the purposes of consistency and authenticity in the delivery of the material, it is important that each course stays true to the approved course objectives.

Building on Prior Knowledge

As faculty members and administrators in sport management look at the macro perspective of our program, we need to be sequential in our course offerings. In addition, we need to be sure students are building on their prior knowledge. A clear progression should be in place and be planned out for students to progressively learn and add to their sport management core knowledge as well as their general core knowledge. Most institutions do have mechanisms in place to ensure students complete, let's say, "SM 100: Introduction to Sport Management" before "SM 220: Sport Marketing." Most colleges and universities also use the designated numbers "100" and "200" level courses as introductory or foundation type courses. Then, students in their third and fourth years will complete upper level courses where there is higher level critical thinking and application to their internships or practical experiences and building in relations to the theories conceived in the lower level or foundations courses.

Course Activities: Issues of Consistency and Duplication

Often, several faculty members in our academic programs teach the same course. Whether the courses are offered in the same semester or not, the importance of the consistent use of activities and learning outcomes cannot be overstated. To document the learning progress of all sport management students by course and by year in the program, sport management educators should plan for the delivery of course objectives, the use of the same course rubrics for assignments, similar tests and exams, and consistent readings and assignments. In conducting outcomes assessment, to measure student learning sport management administrators require a consistent evaluation tool or measurement to make comparisons from course to course or from student to student.

Assessment Activities

Each institution varies in the determination of course objectives and activities in each of the sport management courses offered. One important question for sport management educators to explore is this: How do we determine which assessment activities we will include in our courses? Some sport management educators have a programmed slate of courses they teach. As the professor who teaches that course we know what we are doing, and often we assume others within our department know what we are doing. Unfortunately, that is not the case. Too often many sport management professors teaching different courses are at times guilty of assigning the same type of project to students from one class to the next without any thought that the activity has been part of another course. Surely, good teaching ideas seem to be used over and over again.

As programs grow and new faculty members join the department, it is important for an orientation of some sort to occur at the departmental level to ensure that all teaching members, full and part time, are on the "same page." In many programs of study, where accreditation and external approval have been instrumented for decades, a clearinghouse in which academic deans can review the syllabus has been instated. The clearinghouse systematically ensures the course syllabus is clear and accurate, the course objectives are approved, and course projects and assignments are not duplicated from course to course. This attention to detail is essential when we are establishing the delivery a quality sport management program. Professors very often have a sense of ownership with their course, which is a good thing, because we all want sport management educators

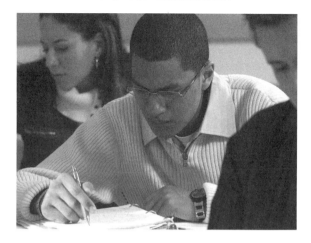

to take pride in their teaching. However, sport management administrators must make sure faculty members are not alone on an island when preparing course content.

It is certainly important that concepts flow from one course to another and that introductory courses teach the fundamental concepts, whereas the upper level courses build and expand on those basic topics. The intent of the sport management program of study is that the courses offered are sequential and progress from introductory or basic to more advanced content topics. If we treat sport management courses as stand-alone works, then students will not reap the benefits of forward-thinking programs. Programs will lack the requisite building blocks, and sport management educators will ultimately fail to develop effective leaders and practitioners in the sport management industry.

Assessment is an ongoing process of understanding and improving student learning. Unfortunately, in education today the final grade has become the focus of students in our courses versus the process of acquiring new skills and learning. The question of how one gets an "A" has been echoed through the halls of colleges and universities for years. Learning assessment takes on two approaches: formative and summative. Simply stated, grades are final and are based on the content created for assignments or examinations. The formative type, on the other hand, takes a more diagnostic or progressive approach to encouraging student learning. Sport management educators can adopt the formative approach to shape their teaching methods in an attempt to improve the quality of student learning. In summary, assessment allows sport management educators to focus on collecting feedback on student acquisition of knowledge and then in turn using that data or information to ultimately improve teaching.

Teaching Tip

Certainly there are many assessment techniques one can use throughout courses to obtain information on how well students understand the concepts we are teaching.

1. *Five-minute drill:* Students indicate in a brief paper the most important things learned through the reading, assignment, or lecture and what issues remain unclear.

2. *Point clarification:* From the lecture or reading, what was the least clear to students? Students can respond in class, through an online forum, or by e-mail.

3. *Concept mapping or tracking:* Students are asked to create a concept map as to what they have learned about topics and connect them. Concept maps allow students to visually connect topics to a central idea. Sport management seniors can create concept maps to connect all the course content in sport management with course concepts in their general education courses or even electives.

4. *Debriefing after a class discussion:* Professors can summarize and highlight key topics and discussion points. Students will be able to synthesize the information and ask follow-up questions when needed.

5. *Pulse of class:* Sport management professors can take some time to ask students about the assignments they are completing and their progress with the work in the course.

6. *Post-test:* Students must be held accountable for the amount of time they spend studying and preparing for test examinations. It is important for sport management professors to probe and ask students the amount of study time devoted to tests. Professors should communicate their expectations regarding the appropriate amount of time that should be allocated to the tested topics.

7. *Class quiz:* Professors can prepare three to five questions relating to the course. The questions can be from past readings, definitions, and case studies. In addition, the questions can also be a window to learning more about the needs of the students enrolled. Professors can ask students to share their feelings about the pace of lectures, the challenges of the course assignments, and provide an overall rating of the course. Mixing course topic questions with feedback type questions provides the sport management educator with rich information regarding students and the course material.

8. *Sample projects:* Students benefit from visually reviewing a project that has been submitted by other students in prior terms or semesters. The students can use the opportunity to get a better sense of the course expectations relating to the project. Students should be

made aware that each term the project requirements may change and that they should use student samples as a model but not to necessarily reproduce the same material.

9. *Test question preparation:* To motivate students to create study habits, students can be assigned to post or e-mail test questions to the professor at designated points throughout the semester. Students will need to spend time constructing questions that are relevant for an examination. Sport management professors can ask students to develop questions after a lecture, in class activity, reading, or guest speaker. The student-created test questions can be shared with the entire class and be used as a study guide.

All of these quick exercises can be adapted to fit specific course needs. The point is that sport management educators must incorporate activities that will tell us whether students are learning or need more clarification.

Engaging Students

Creating a dynamic and energetic classroom must be a goal for all of us who teach in higher education. Sustaining students' passion for learning over a semester is a time-consuming process. At any point in the semester sport management educators can reflect on their efforts of connecting and engaging students. One enlightening piece of research is Gamson and Chickering's "Seven Principles for Good Practice in Undergraduate Education" (1987). Developed from a review of 50 years of educational literature, the seven principles are as follows:

1. Encourages contact between student and faculty
2. Develops reciprocity and cooperation among students
3. Encourages active learning
4. Gives prompt feedback
5. Emphasizes time on task
6. Communicates high expectations
7. Respects diverse talents and ways of learning

As sport management educators read over these principles, they can serve as a guide in teaching. Through a closer examination when each principle is simplified and broken down, sport management educators can make connections to their teaching methodology, their interactions with students, and communication with students on an individual level and within the formal class structure.

Encourages Contact Between Students and Faculty

In the sport management industry many of our programs of study require students to complete practical and/or internship experiences. Very often, students rely on the contacts that a professor has in a particular field

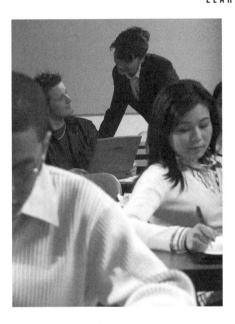

or rely on the professor's knowledge about specific sport businesses and organizations. Building a rapport, especially in such a changing and dynamic field, is an important ingredient, not only in good teaching but in building a high-level program. Mentoring has always been a "buzz word" on college campuses. Transferring a mentoring system to the courses sport management educators teach can propel some students who would often hide in the back of the class to become more active in the course.

Teaching Tip

For the online arena contact between students and professors takes on a different but similar dimension. Online educators can still tap into the benefits of this principle. The design of the course should allow for interactions. Discussion boards can be used to ask students to communicate areas of interest and future employment opportunities and to communicate and connect with students. Some software programs allow virtual office hours: Although the student may not be sitting in front of you in your office, you still have designated time to devote to building contacts with students and helping them navigate their way through the course, the sport management program, or with other academic issues and concerns.

Develops Reciprocity and Cooperation Among Students

Team building has been part of coaching philosophies for decades. Adding a team building model to courses mirrors what occurs in the workplace and can create healthy relationships and dynamics within the classroom environment. Using the team-building concept is useful in teaching, because we get a group of individuals on day 1 and we need them to all be working together at some level and toward a common goal by day 7. We have 6 days to have each student have some interaction with other students in class. This model assists in building "class chemistry" that students appreciate, especially in the first semester when getting to know the rest of the students in the major may be difficult. With those team-building activities the class can then build a "classroom culture" where the group has an understanding of what is acceptable academic behavior and what are the expectations of the group. Students can work together at setting higher standards when considering this guiding philosophy. Sport management is an industry where we must work with others in small units or in larger working groups. An educational introduction to that is to foster an environment where students value and respect working with others.

Encourages Active Learning

If educators could construct their own classroom, how many rows of seats would we create? From the author's perspective, I have always believed there should only be one row in a college course—the front row. The "front rowers" must always be on their toes ready for the next question, always looking prepared, and always taking notes. So, how do sport management educators find ways to get the rest of the class involved? Simply put, educators must teach and encourage learning. Sport management educators must incorporate teaching cues to get students involved whether it is calling on a student randomly or setting up activities that promote student contributions to course discussions. Inactive learning encourages students to just sit in class and write notes word for word. Active educators incorporate and embed discussion questions within lectures to promote open discussion and higher order thinking skills.

A revealing question typically incorporated in many course evaluations is the amount of time students spend studying/preparing for the course outside of the designated class time. One suggestion can be that those students in a 50-minute class that meets three times a week need to spend at least 3 hours a week completing class activities/studying on their own time. Sport management educators must be committed to fostering an environment whereby students are accountable for being self-learners. It is important that sport management professors do not perform all the work in a sense through their delivery of the course content or by hand feeding the students with information. A dynamic classroom environment is invigorating, and students become active contributors and create a sense of ownership within the course discussions. The professor can, in fact, facilitate learning as the students begin to share and explore their experiences and research within the classroom setting. This type of atmosphere fosters a rich learning environment.

Teaching Tip

In the classroom, include activities that will be part of the lecture. These activities encourage student participation, they become part of the lecture, and then the notes become real and practical in sport management lives. Staying current in the topics and issues of sport management also assists in building a dynamic class environment.

Teaching Tip

For online educators, all of these students are indeed in the first row. Students by the nature of online educators must all be active in the courses because they need to be "seen" by the professor by contributing to blogs and discussion boards.

Gives Prompt Feedback

Prompt feedback is not always easy when many sport management professors have large teaching loads and multiple sections of courses. However, it is important to strive to return student work with comments, affirmations, and strategies for improvement as soon as possible.

Emphasizes Time on Task

Students live busy lives and have difficulty balancing their social and personal activities with their academic pursuits. Students are often enrolled in four or five courses each term or semester. To complete their work at a high level and on time, simple mechanisms can be put in place by sport management educators to assist students (**Box 1.1**).

BOX (1.1) Recommendations for Students.

1. Use a daily planner and plot course assignments and due dates.
2. Plan in advance; do not wait until the last moment to complete an assignment.
3. Review the syllabus often to be sure the course content and material are understood.
4. Discuss any issues with time management with your professor.

Sport management educators can set a level of classroom expectations for students to comply. Creating a "classroom corporate culture" gives students a clear understanding of the accepted behaviors in the college classroom.

Teaching Tip

Treat students like sport management professional. Indicate that each classroom session is a meeting for the workplace. Encourage students to arrive early and begin preparing for the current day's topic. Many times, students need reminding that the class is a common location shared by many people. Late arrivals or class disturbances cannot occur because they disrupt the flow of the class.

Communicates High Expectations

Often, creating a course with challenges becomes a double-edged sword for many professors. Rigor can at times be confused with too much work. There is certainly a fine line. Students do evaluate faculty members, and at times it becomes a popularity contest. Typically, professors who are more lenient or considered to be "easy graders" very often receive praise. Sport management educators must continue to challenge students in the classroom because ultimately they are representatives of the institution. Students often respond to educators who encourage them to exceed expectations. Professors can incorporate a variety of motivational techniques to encourage sport management students to strive to excel in courses.

Teaching Tip

Through course activities students can get an awareness and accurate sense of what it will be like in the "real world." Sport management educators can be diligent in expressing classroom expectations in the course syllabus. Very often a professor will get a reputation of being tough—take that as a compliment!

Respects Diverse Talents and Ways of Learning

Educators today are aware of the diverse needs of our learners. It is certainly important for educators to tap into those skill sets that students are comfortable expressing, it is also our role to teach students new skill sets to allow them to grow and function in the sport management industry. Many faculty members do incorporate a medley or variety of assessment and evaluation tools to assist students on their quest to achieve "good grades" in a course.

Online Instruction: Using the Seven Principles

Frequent contact with students is an important factor in student motivation and involvement. Sport management educators can connect with students online through virtual office hours and chats and through e-mail to respond to questions and provide direction. If many students have concerns, we can also post a response on the course management system to respond to questions.

Technology also provides instructors with another tool to have students work in groups, whether it is in the form of a partnership, debate, or even students who are expert presenters on their research topic, and other students can provide feedback. Technology can make all students sit in the front row. When assignments and activities are moved online students become active learners. Students cannot expect the professor to entertain them and fill 50 minutes of time with lecture. Students become accountable for their own learning.

Current sport management educators may recognize that the way they were taught in higher education is not the same as it is today. In the modern-day classroom sport management educators and educators in general have become more focused on creating critical thinkers, innovators, and lifelong learners. Although there is certainly a time and a place for the utilization of lectures and reading materials, sport management educators can continue to actively engage students in the learning process and to close the gap between instruction and student learning so the process becomes seamless by using web-enhanced technologies in courses. In the learner-centered environment professors are actively involved in ensuring students are "getting it" and that the concepts are clear and comprehended by students. In the learner-centered environment, students believe that faculty members are concerned with their learning and that professors are paying attention to their needs. As a result, students become more motivated to achieve in those settings. The concept of learning to learn is central to creating a dynamic and interactive course environment.

Teaching Tip

Many times students have questions relating to course content that has been reviewed multiple times in a class. To promote student thinking and self-learning we can encourage students to ask three of their course mates before seeking the help of the professor—ask three before me! Often, students can discover a solution by collaborating versus getting a simple scripted response of how to earn an A.

Integrating Technology Tools

Embarking on incorporating technology and web-enhanced tools into your teaching may seem like a daunting task. The "buzz word" when technology is the topic on hand is integration. Instructors should focus on how technology can improve the learning environment. Ensuring that the integration of technology use is for the benefit and not the detriment of classroom learning is the key to teaching effectively with these new media tools. As we reflect back to the use of e-mail, many skeptics existed in academia. Many never believed that the use of e-mail would become a, if not the, primary practice of communication between professors and students. Additionally, the World Wide Web has connected educators and students alike to the world and beyond. Information (accurate or not) is literally at the touch of our fingertips.

Guide to Incorporating Technology Into the Sport Management Curriculum

Many college campuses are being outfitted with remarkable abilities to deliver state-of-the-art teaching classrooms. Perhaps many sport management educators are feeling the pressure to keep up with the technologically advances. To continue to effectively teach in the sport management program of study, sport management educators can use the following guide:

1. Technology becomes part of your teaching. To enhance your teaching using technology, be sure the enhancements used become part of the structure of your teaching plans versus stand-alone concepts. Students and faculty members alike need to feel comfortable with the injection of technology or web-enhanced activities within the classroom environment. The integration of technology needs to be connected to your delivery of course content and not just used because of the pressure to add technology to the teaching classroom.

2. Technology has a purpose within your course structure. One essential force behind incorporating technology into the classroom is to be sure there is a plan for its use throughout the semester. Sport management students need to be exposed to technology and web-enhanced activities in a comfortable learning setting. Sport management educators must find the effective balance between traditional teaching and teaching with technology.

3. Technology is the tool; the professor is the carpenter! We all need to recognize that sport management educators who use technology in the classroom need to understand its value and purpose. Using technology just for the sake of it will not leave

a positive impression on the students in the class. At the onset of initiating technology into the classroom, sport management educators may want to use tools they are most familiar and comfortable using. Over time, adding new tools to the teaching toolbox will make more sense rather than incorporating multiple technologies without a true sense of the value of the medium.

New Territory: Web-Enhanced Courses

Throughout the process of moving into a new way of thinking by creating technology or web-enhanced courses, it has become apparent that some sport management faculty members are uncomfortable with the use of technology. Many questions need to be addressed by sport management educators when deciding to implement a technology initiative into courses. One central question is whether there is a system of support for sport management faculty members who need assistance integrating new media into the classroom delivery. In many of our academic departments we have an informal technology mentor who assists others with troubleshooting technology issues. One way to create a seamless transition with integration of technology throughout a 4-year program of study is to designate a formal technology mentor. The technology mentor should be a person with whom most faculty members feel a level of comfort and security. Perhaps the technology mentor could also receive a course reduction to support the needs of others in the sport management department.

Transitioning to a web-enhanced approach to teaching is a time-consuming initiative that can be met with some resistance if the teaching and learning benefits are not clearly communicated to all the vested parties. The process can become the "survival of the technologically fit." Sport management academic administrators must be aware and concerned that some faculty members may be left behind. In addition, sport management educators need to be sure that the lack of technology use in courses would not lead to consequences in class evaluations, merit, or tenure.

How can we support the needs of sport management faculty members while promoting the use of technology in the classroom? This is where sport management programs can collaborate with other faculty members on campus whose majors have already moved forward in the technology initiative. Cultivating academic relationships with colleagues across disciplines can assist in making the transition to teaching with technology. A variety of course structures currently exists as viable options for sport management educators to consider when creating courses and course contest (**Box 1.2**).

BOX (1.2) Types of Teaching Classrooms Utilizing Technology

- *Web-enhanced courses:* Web-enhanced courses are often connected to traditional classrooms that incorporate activities requiring the use of materials from the Internet or program software. In addition, web-enhanced courses may also rely on the use of the college course management system.
- *Course management systems:* Course management systems are typically housed within our institutional computer systems. There are many variations of course management systems, such as Web Ct, Blackboard, and many others. These programs allow instructors to post syllabi, readings, and discussion board questions and to embed technology within their courses.
- *Hybrid courses:* Typical hybrid courses incorporate traditional face-to-face teaching combined with courses held completely online. Hybrid courses provide a new twist to the traditional lecture courses of the past. Sport management educators have the opportunity to explore course concepts during designated meeting times throughout the term, while also allowing students to discover knowledge and present information utilizing a variety of technologies or course management systems from their own desktop. The value and appeal of hybrid courses rests with the combination of both online and face-to-face activities.
- *Online courses:* The delivery of an entire course from start to finish conducted solely from the sport management educator's computer to student computer is considered an online course. Thus online courses have led to the term "virtual classroom," which can be defined as any online opportunity where students and professors "connect" and "exchange ideas" utilizing their desktop computers.

Sport management programs and educators need to look at educational technology as a tool to enhance student learning. Educational technology can be looked at as building interactive activities into sport management courses. Gilbert and Moore (1998) defined interaction as a "reciprocal exchange between the technology and the learner which in turn promotes and encourages feedback and discourse and active participation in the learning process" (p. 31). One central concern of many faculty members when considering offering hybrid or online courses is how to make the learner feel connected or part of the learning process. An academic experience that is both enriching and challenging can be created through virtual classrooms and learning environments based on both hybrid and online courses where participants (faculty members and students) never or rarely meet.

Surely, the "human element" needs to be included in our courses even when we add the technology component to our courses. Effective educators must still listen, respond, and probe.

Teaching Tip

Integrating technology can be a significant asset to learners in the classroom. Evaluate your courses:

- Where can you use or integrate educational technology?
- Where can educational technology improve student acquisition of knowledge?
- How can educational technology resources support student learning?

Although incorporating technology and web-enhanced features to sport management courses is important, equally important is determining the level of technology use and ability of students. Sport management educators and program administrators can survey students at the start and end of the semester to determine the actual use and student comfort with technology and educational software.

Teaching Tip

Survey students to determine what changes need to be made to deliver a more effective course. How often do our students use technology:

- For course activities?
- To access course information and content on course websites?
- To access library resources or materials posted on course management systems?
- To complete an in-class or out-of-class assignments?
- For creating presentations?
- For creating websites or computer-generated graphics?

Questions to Consider

- What works and what does not work in the delivery of your course content?
- What can we learn from our students?
- How can we cultivate faculty mentoring programs to help each other navigate through the technology maze?
- How can we develop learning outcomes from the integration of technology into the classroom?
- How can we reflect and evaluate the use of technology that is incorporated in a course to determine its effectiveness in the learning process?

R e f e r e n c e s

Commission on Sport Management Accreditation (COSMA). (2008). Accreditation Principles and Self Study Preparation. Available at: http://iweb.aahperd.org/naspe/cosma/pdf_files/ accrPrinciples.pdf. Accessed April 2, 2009.

Davis, K. A. (1994). *Sport management: Successful private sector business strategies.* Madison, WI: Brown & Benchmark.

Fielding, L. W., Pitts, B. G., & Miller, L. K. (1991). Defining quality: Why should educators in sport management be concerned about quality? *Journal of Sport Management, 5*(1):1–17.

Gamson, Z. F., & Chickering, A. W. (1987). Seven principles for good practice in undergraduate education. *AAHE Bulletin,* March, 5–10.

Gilbert, L., & Moore, D. R. (1998). Building interactivity into web courses: Tools for social and instructional interaction. *Educational Technology,* 38(3), 29–35.

Laird, C. (2005). The influence of sport management program characteristics in academician's perceptions of NASPE-NASSM approval. *SMART Online Journal,* 1(2), 1–13.

National Association of Sport and Physical Education-North American Society for Sport Management [NASPE-NASSM]. (2000). *Sport management program standards and review protocol.* Reston, VA: Author.

National Association of Sport and Physical Education-North American Society for Sport Management [NASPE-NASSM]. (2007). *COSMA accreditation manual.* Reston, VA: Author.

Parkhouse, B. L., & Pitts, B. G. (2001). Definition, evolution, and curriculum. In B. L. Parkhouse (Ed.), *The management of sport* (pp. 2–14). New York: McGraw-Hill.

Pitts, B. G. (2001). Sport management at the millennium: A defining moment. *Journal of Sport Management,* 15(1), 1–9.

Pitts, B., & Stotlar, D. (2002). *Fundamentals of sport marketing.* Morgantown, WV: Fitness Information Technologies.

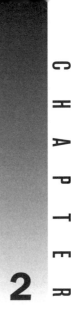

Teaching Activities: Foundation of Sport Management

A number of institutions incorporate a first-level or introductory course into the sport management major. Through experience and research it is apparent that sport management educators spend a large amount of time working with students in the areas of internship and career exploration in these courses. In addition, basic managerial functions, roles, and responsibilities are also explored in this entry-level or introductory course into the major. The course topics and activities in this chapter can be easily implemented to guide students in the process of discovering what sport management means to their future endeavors, first as a student and then as a sport management professional. The following content areas are explored in this chapter:

- Sport leadership
- Sport management internships and careers
- Strategic planning
- Resume writing and the interview process

Sport Leadership

Activity I: Sport Management Interest Group Formation

Students form working groups in the traditional classroom setting or online from their personal computer. The groups are established by the interests the students have in the field. For instance, students interested in sport marketing will form a group, those with an inclination in athletic administration will form a group, and those interested in sport law will form a group. The groups begin their journey by exchanging names and contact information. The second task of the groups is to assign themselves a team name that reflects their sport management interests along with the personalities of the individuals forming the group. Once the team name is established, the groups must adopt a slogan or motto that serves as their motivation throughout the course.

The entire class learns about the intent of each group and names of group members. Students begin to share ideas and appreciate the diversity of others in the larger classroom setting. Bonds and connections are secured through a simple activity that may take 10 to 15 minutes to develop. These groups can remain intact, and they can be called on to complete group projects and assignments in an organized fashion throughout the term.

This icebreaker activity (**Box 2.1**) can be used for a traditional course or online course. Students locate and link with students who have their same passion and connect on a mission of naming the group and creating

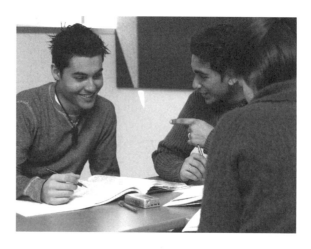

a slogan. Once all groups have completed the initial start-up tasks the information is shared with the entire class. This is a proven and motivational method to connect the small working groups with the entire class.

BOX (2.1) Icebreaker Defined

An icebreaker uses small activities or games to assist in formulating relationships between students. Forming small working units allows students to familiarize themselves with others in larger groups and build safe environments for growth, learning, and sharing of ideas and information.

Activity II: Effective Management and Leadership

Early in this course students can be encouraged to think like sport managers or sport administrators. To engage the students and allow them to critically analyze decisions of sport business professionals, we can present lecture material and theoretical information on leadership. Sport management educators, for example, can begin this activity with definitions of leadership, what constitutes leadership in an organization, which personal attributes contribute to good leadership, and contemporary research regarding sport leadership.

For an assignment all students are to select one leader (unfamiliar to the masses) in sport management or a corporate setting. Next, students select one personal leader who has made an impact on their lives. Each student finds an article depicting the sport management leader, describing his or her role in the industry, how he or she influenced or changed his or her particular segment of the sport management industry, and what the student learned from this person. In addition, students write a portrait depicting the influential personal leader and what they have gained from their experience with that person. Students must then synthesize their work into a written document expressing their perspective on leadership, characteristics they most value from the selected leaders, and how they would like people to describe them as a leader in sport management 15 years from now.

Teaching Tip

Students can post the information they have collected for this assignment online. Students can be creative and add stories, photos, or links to the works of these selected leaders. Students, within a discussion board or forum, can conduct a "Questions and Answers" session as it relates to their selections. This collaborative piece of the assignment allows students to actively engage one another free of any prompting by the professor.

Activity III: Successful Managers

Most, if not all, sport management students in our classes have held previous employment positions. Through those experiences students have obtained knowledge regarding managers and management in a variety of settings. Even if these experiences are outside of the sport management domain, students acquire a rich sense of what it is like to be an employee, the decisions managers make on a daily basis, the interaction and dynamics of the workplace, and the different personalities of senior management. Through those workplace experiences students derive a profile of what constitutes successful and unsuccessful management. The lessons learned from practical experiences transfers into insightful classroom discourse.

For the classroom activity students can list the positive and negative attributes of a manager they have experienced in the work setting. If by chance students have no workplace experience, they can tap into their athletic experiences and contribute using coaches as substitute managers. Once the individual list is created, students can form a partnership with a course mate. Students then discuss any variations from the list. The sport management professor can lead a discussion on management theory, such as scientific management, management science, classical approaches to management, and the behavioral approach. In addition, the sport management educator can share information regarding the background and motivation of the founders and scientists who developed each approach. From the lectures and practical experiences students can then critically analyze which type of leadership attributes they wish to develop as future sport managers. Students have the capability to distinguish between effective and ineffective management through these exercises.

Teaching Tip

Students can write about their personal and professional experiences with diverse management styles in a course blog. Comments are required to focus on both the positive and negative aspects of each theory. Students create links to pertinent articles, information, and current event stories that can be included to fully develop the blog chatter.

Activity IV: Current Leaders in the Sport Management Industry

Various trade and professional journals publish information on top-ranked leaders in sport business. The names and faces of these influential people may not be as recognizable as the athletes and sports they have successful molded, but their stories are terrific learning opportunities for our students. Students are asked to pick one person off that list to research and share with the class. Students are very often surprised with the discovery of information. Students can emulate "real people" in the industry and appreciate the diverse backgrounds and education of these professionals.

Often, we learn about leadership from our parents, teachers, or coaches. We learn about leaders through stories and movies. As sport management majors students start to critically analyze the decisions leaders must make in business and athletic arenas. Encouraging students to closely examine leaders in the industry of sport business can be an eye-opening experience. As students progress through their courses, their perspective on issues may change, as will their perspective of leadership in the sport management setting. This early launch to studying leadership in the first semester or year in the program sets the stage as students look to gain meaningful internships and volunteer experiences where leadership is emphasized and stressed. Students also have the chance in class or through an online discussion board to share and discuss their leadership selections.

Teaching Tip

For use in a traditional or online course, professors can require students to post the name of a sport business industry leader and find one more article to link and share with the class.

Activity V: Campus Leaders in Sport and Athletics

Invite campus leaders in the sport management arena to share their perspectives with the class. Campus members such as the Athletic Director, Facility Manager, Aquatics Director, Intramural Coordinator, Athletic Coaches, and Athletic Trainer can all be valuable to classroom discussions. Sport management professors can coordinate an "Ask the Expert" session throughout the semester or term. These connections with campus leaders, especially for first-year students, create enriching bonds. Seasoned professionals can share their inspirational leadership stories and accounts with the class. In addition, these professionals can share their personal athletic administration journeys with the field with the group. Students can write a summary reflection piece that synthesizes the materials from the presentations and their own research.

Internships and Careers

Activity I: Internship Discovery

One of the first questions prospective and enrolled students ask revolves around internship and career opportunities in sport management. For this activity instructors can discuss the segments of the sport management industry along with the long list of possible career opportunities in sport business. Students can determine which segment is the best fit for their first internship or area of concentration. The umbrella that is sport management covers so many diverse and interesting career opportunities. As a sport management educator it is our role to serve as a guide to systematically assist students in exploring the segments of the sport management industry that they find most appealing. In addition, sport management educators need to be familiar with and comfortable in providing information about the particulars of those career paths.

At many institutions students are required to complete various internships at various points in their academic career. To systematically guide students instructors can use benchmarks throughout the semester to "check in" (**Table 2.1**) on student progress toward their discovery of potential internship sites. The written activity presented in Table 2.1 can be submitted on paper or electronically through electronic portfolio or online course management systems. Instructors can determine the length of the information that needs to be submitted along with the proper timeline for due dates.

Table 2.1 Check-In Benchmarks

Check-In Part I
- List three possible internship sites.
- List the internship contact person in the organization.
- List the responsibilities of an intern at these sites.

Check-In Part II
Select two organizations from the original list.
- Under which segment(s) of the sport management industry do these organizations fall?
- Describe the organizations' core markets.
- What career opportunities are available to you?
- Summarize two articles relating to these organizations.
- Indicate if these organizations are profit or nonprofit.
- What is their mission statement?
- List the changes over the last 2 years or last 10 years.
- List the short-term plans of the organization.
- List the long-term plans of the organization.
- Provide a sample cover letter to be sent to one organization.

Check-In Part III
Narrow focus to one organization.
- Size of organization
  - Number of employees
  - Presence of subdivisions

- Detailed mission statement
  - Type of company (products/services)
  - Future direction of company
  - What makes the company unique
- Organizational objectives
- Organization strategies (market penetration and one other)
- Article summary for organization
- Industry competitors

Activity II: Internship Poster Presentation or Virtual Poster Presentation

Once students have had the opportunity to research and study sport organizations, the next step is to share the collected information with course mates. For traditional face-to-face classes instructors can organize a poster presentation session not unlike the sessions we experience at academic conferences. For hybrid or online courses instructors can require students to post a visual or virtual poster and allow course mates to post follow-up questions through a designated discussion board or forum for an allotted period of time. Poster presentations are acceptable means of presenting and sharing information and research in professional associations; therefore the value of this type of assessment activity stretches into the professional realm as well. Poster presentations can be used in a variety of courses, and students like the divergence from the typical in class presentation. Poster presentations allow students to think creatively and share their work in a face-to-face or one-on-one format instead of one student addressing a class of 25 of their peers. Expectations of the poster presentations should be made clear to the students for consistency in the process. In fact, the list can be transformed into a rubric for grading purposes (**Table 2.2**).

Table 2.2 Poster Presentation Guidelines

1. Clearly write the company name.
2. Use creative photos, slogans, and mission statements to attract an audience to your poster.
3. The poster should tell the audience about the company and you (from a sport management perspective).
4. You are the expert for the company. Provide as much information as possible on the poster.
5. You must have prepared statements about the company and your role as an intern. We will be asking questions.

Activity III: Portfolio Reflection—Internship Discovery

Before the availability of electronic portfolio software, many in higher education used a simple folder method by which students housed important and designated materials for a course. This activity can be in either format to suit the needs of the instructor or program of study. The questions in **Table 2.3** are presented to students for response. The nature of the questions are such that students demonstrate their growth and learning in the area of internship and career path discovery very early in their academic careers. The questions presented in Table 2.3 can be incorporated into an electronic or hard-copy portfolio types.

The internship project is a critical and important focus of the curriculum. Encouraging students to reflect on the process of discovering internship sites and to communicate and share how the journey has transformed or confirmed their passion in the sport management industry relates specifically to outcome assessment in sport management education. Perhaps students have changed their focus a bit more once they uncover certain aspects about one particular sector of the industry. Typically, this process of internship discovery is an affirmation of the student's desire to

Table 2.3 Sport Management Portfolio Checklist

- Discuss the three places you considered for the project. What factors about the companies most appealed to you?
- Compare the two mission statements developed in Table 2.1, Check-In Part II. Are they effective? What changes would you make? Do the statements motivate workers?
- How did the articles collected for the check-ins help you learn more about the sport management industry?
- What sector of the industry (based on your research) would you feel most comfortable working under? Why?
- From Table 2.1, Check-In Part III, and Table 2.2, what company did you choose? Why was it more appealing to you than the other two?
- What opportunities are available to you or a sport manager at that company?
- How are the company mission statements different from each other? Compare and contrast collected check-ins?
- How have the check-ins helped you to find internship opportunities and/or learn more about sport management?
- Would you recommend any changes to the project?

---

pursue a particular segment of the sport management industry. For most students the internship process is a large component of their 4-year program of study. The Internship Process Guide (**Table 2.4**) can be a checklist of activities that students complete to facilitate learning about potential internship sites and steps to secure the opportunity.

Table 2.4 Internship Process Guide

- *Search and information collection:* By requiring internship check-ins students will have detailed information regarding three sport organizations along with contact information and potential opportunities.
- *Role of intern:* Before committing to a sport organization, students must be sure to discuss their role as an intern with the structure of the organization. It is helpful if the organization has worked with the institution in the past or has at least supervised interns from other institutions. Students who do not formally pinpoint their role in the organization may select an internship that leaves them completing tasks that are not educational or enriching.
- *Contact with sport organization:* Before any contact with potential internship sites, students must be made aware of the appropriate protocol for contacting professionals over the phone and/or through e-mail correspondence. Practice makes perfect in this area. Students who practice their communication and interviewing skills are better off in these situations than those students who attempt to "cold contact" internship sites.
- *Selection:* Students need to be sure to select an internship site that meets their professional goals and can reach their learning objectives for the program of study. Students can be guided to select internship sites that enrich and compliment their academic studies.
- *Debrief:* Once the internship experience is complete and all required hours are logged, students need the opportunity to share their experiences with others. The power of debriefing after an internship experience is twofold: students get a chance to share with others all their accomplishments and growth through the internship, and the other students get a chance to listen and learn from course mates. Debriefing sessions expose students to new opportunities and allows students to highlight their professional achievements in the sport management industry.
- *Look ahead:* Once an internship is complete students should be encouraged to think about their next opportunity within the field. Students should also be sure to remain in contact with the professionals they worked with in previous settings to stay in touch with the industry and future opportunities.

The process of research and discovery of internship information is practical and important in the minds and lives of sport management students. Sport management students realize the importance of finding and securing internships; therefore these projects become a delight for students and a central focus for their academic career.

Strategic Planning

A variety of courses may include the topic of strategic planning or some components of strategic planning. Some courses that incorporate the topic can be Introduction to Sport Management, Sport Marketing, Sport Finance and Economics, Sport in the Global Marketplace, and Organization of Sport Businesses.

Activity I: Sport Business Research

Sport management educators can organize students into work groups. An effective group size is three to four students. If instructors have established groups for other activities, students can remain in pre-established group designated during the course, or new teams can be created. Before the start of the course the instructor researches five to six sport organizations. The sport-related companies allow students to apply their knowledge on strategic planning. Examples of companies can be Gatorade (parent company, PepsiCo, Inc.), Under Armour, Nike, Schwinn Bicycles, or Boston College. Sport management educators can be creative in selecting the companies or organizations.

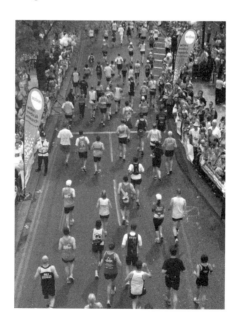

Teaching Tip

In some instances the use of a lottery process has helped level the playing field in selecting a company to work with. One team captain selects an index card randomly placed along the desktop. Students typically hem and haw if they don't get a particular organization; this adds to the energy in the class. Once each group has a company, the strategic planning process begins.

Stages of the Strategic Planning Process

The first piece of the project is for students to bring into class current and topical articles about their designated company. Students must have different information than the others in their group. This encourages students to communicate with one another outside designated class time. Next, students meet in their groups to share their information with the class. It becomes an interesting dynamic when students are empowered to share the information.

Teaching Tip

At the start of the assignment, students are made well aware that they are executives in the company trying to provide a new direction to an existing company in the marketplace. From prior experience students take true ownership in the project when they believe they have a stake in the outcome.

Strategic Planning Benchmark Assignments

1. Discovery of current information as it relates to designated company. Students locate information about their designated company by using the library database or Internet search engines.
2. Creation of mission statement based on existing company objectives. Some of the selected companies may or may not have a published website. For the companies that do provide the general public with their mission statement, students can indicate the strengths and weaknesses in that document and suggest changes. For companies without a mission statement, students create a statement that reflects the companies past accomplishments, present directions, and future goals.
3. Creation of clear objectives. One aspect of the strategic planning process is to develop objectives for sport organizations that are

specific and measurable. Students must determine the direction and goals of the company and create three objectives.

4. Creation of strategies (market penetration, market development, product development, and diversification). Using the four strategies within the strategic planning process, students communicate the target market(s) and product/services the company will offer to reach stated goals and company objectives.

5. Organizational chart. Within this topic instructors can spend time discussing power and authority within the chain of command of the designated companies. Students can determine which hierarchy they are working with and which chain of command they would use if they were an executive at those companies. Additionally, instructors can include a lecture on professional job descriptions. Students can then research the specific roles and responsibilities of company staff. Students are also exposed to the professional job titles they may encounter in the industry as they research internship and career opportunities.

6. Future direction of company. Under this section students can apply their critical thinking skills and start to use the collected information to forecast the future direction for the company. Should the company expand their product line? Should the company get more or less involved with collegiate or professional sport? Sport management educators can start to pose some interesting questions, and students can then become decision makers for a sport organization.

7. Movers and shakers within the company. Students begin to learn more about the personnel in the company. If the students can access the educational backgrounds of the company executives, they may become more motivated in their quest to complete their degree.

Group Presentation

Once the students have invested their time and effort in researching and collecting current information on the company, they will feel a sense of pride and accomplishment in sharing their work with others.

Teaching Tip

For online courses, students can use PowerPoint or a podcast to determine the interesting facts and figures they have learned from the project.

Teaching Tip
For traditional face-to-face courses, instructors can ask students to be creative in the presentations or provide a guide for the type of information and the mode of delivery to the class.

Resume Writing
Often, students who are in the first 2 years of a sport management program do not have a wealth of appropriate experiences to include on a professional resume. At this stage students can collaborate to share honest and open opinions regarding the professional resume. Students can exchange ideas and formats for which resume style is more effective and appropriate for the sport management industry.

Activity I: Who Am I?
To provide assistance in resume development, students start to discuss their personal strengths and weaknesses in the field of sport management. Students have a partner to share their interests and experiences to be include in the professional resume. Through this exploratory conversation students gain feedback while also providing insightful details to other students.

Activity II: Feedback
At this stage students would have a chance to submit a draft of their current resume. Some first-year students fail to update their educational data. Students are asked to submit their resume to three other students in the class. Each student then has a collection of three other opinions and suggestions for enhancing and improving the resume. At the same time each student also acts as a reader of three other resumes. This process fosters respect and appreciation of the work of others and allows students to be active contributors for this important in-class assignment.

Activity III: Revisions
Once students have had the chance to read and synthesize the comments of others, they work on submitting a new and improved resume for grading. Students are prompted to include the comments of the reviewers along with the new resume copy. The professor can ascertain the changes that have occurred to the resume while reviewing the comments of at least three other students along with the final version.

Activity IV: Interview Questions
Students are prompted to create a list of potential questions the internship/career site will ask candidates in an interview setting. Students then

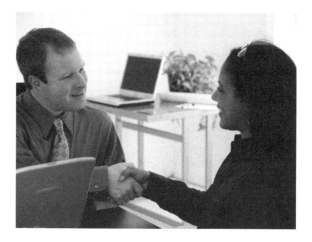

share lists with one another and discuss their content. Professors can then lead a discussion regarding the interview format and expectations. Dress code and appropriate body language skill development can also be incorporated into the activity. The next step is for students to consider a list of questions they would ask the company committee members during or after the interview process. Students should gain an understanding of why it is important to ask follow-up questions in this type of setting.

Activity V: The Interview
Students interview one another by using the previously created list of questions. Student interviewees submit a job description so the student interviewer can use that document during the "Questions and Answers" activity. The students have time to interview one another and to critique each other's performance from the welcome handshake to the ending greeting.

The foundation courses in sport management can be the springboard that propels students into the more advanced courses in the program of study. The earlier sport management faculty can engage and connect with students, the more success we will have in preparing successful managers in the industry.

Questions to Consider

- Which teaching methods are you currently incorporating into your course activities that enhance the learning process?
- What other key concepts need to be embedded into a first-year or entry-level sport management course?
- How can you mentor students in their quest to secure educationally sound internships in this competitive sport business environment?

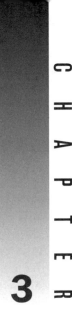

Teaching Activities: Sport Organization Management and Administration

A topical area in sport management is the study of the administration of sport programming at colleges and universities. Some sport management programs may offer a separate stand-alone course in this area or include and embed the principles of this topic within another course. This chapter discusses the following central themes for course content in the area of sport organizational management and administration:

- Comprehensive review of current issues in athletic administration (college, high school, and amateur levels)
- Identification and understanding of the competencies of athletic administrators
- Acquisition of knowledge regarding various methods of budgeting and purchasing

Sport Organization Management and Administration

Activity I: Formation of Institution

To simulate real-world decisions made by athletic administrators, students complete a comprehensive semester-long project that addresses components of athletic management (**Table 3.1**). To begin the semester-long project, students need to develop background and general information regarding their academic and athletic institution they will be creating. The first step in this process is to name the institution and provide a location (city and state). Typically, students are asked to select a location in a specific region to satisfy future requirements of joining a conference and team travel. Once the students select an original name and specific location, students are then asked to select school colors and create a mascot.

Activity II: Conference Affiliation

Next, students are asked to join with a group of students to form an athletic conference. Sport management educators must use their discretion as groups are formed, asking students to shuffle and reshuffle to ensure an appropriate and effective group/conference is created. Depending on the size of the class, students should be in a conference with four and no more than six course mates.

Table 3.1 Sport Scheduling

- Facility planning
- Trouble shooting
- Policy development
- Tournament creation, structure, policies, bracket development
- Budgetary considerations
- Gender equity and Title IX issues
- Contest management: planning for home and away events
- Hiring process and procedures

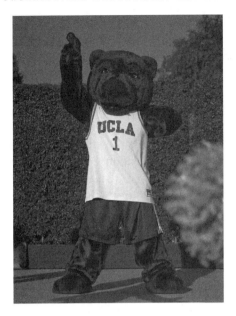

Once the conference is formed, students then work on naming the conference and selecting conference colors. After that exercise students determine conference officials for the semester. Roles may include conference commissioner, conference assistant commissioner, conference secretary, conference web development, and conference corresponding secretary. Students are encouraged to keep meeting minutes for a required four formally created conference meetings.

Activity III: Mission Statement Development

To get a better sense of the direction and purpose of an athletic organization, students are asked to study actual mission statements from Division I, II, and III athletic departments. As an assignment students are asked to select three athletic department mission statements to analyze and share with course mates. Students extract important and meaningful terms and phrases from the existing mission statements. Then, students are required to compare and contrast the mission statements they have collected. In addition, sport management professors can lead a lively discussion relating to the differences of Division I, II, and III National Collegiate Athletic Association (NCAA) member institutions, similarities and distinctions between large and small institutions, and a comprehensive review of athletic departments' purpose in regards to offering athletics to men and women on their college or university campuses.

The second stage in the mission statement activity is for students to develop and write a mission specific to the athletic department they are currently planning to create. Typical mission statements take a volume of work and collaboration from many stakeholders on a college campus. To simulate the process of mission statement development over a much shorter period of time, students are asked to write a two-paragraph (8–10 sentences) mission statement that captures the essence of their athletic department. Once the first draft of the mission statement is written, students share their work with three other people. The selection of reviewers can be students, roommates, other professors, or family members. Each student has three individuals review and critique their mission statement. Based on the feedback collected, students then re-create the mission statement, taking into consideration the comments of others. The mission statement along with the revisions and comments made by the reviewer are all submitted to the professor. The professor has an opportunity to gage the amount of analysis and critical engagement that occurred through the exercise. More revisions may be made based on the remarks of the sport management professor.

The purpose of this activity is twofold. First, sport management students have the opportunity to study the mission statements used by actual athletic departments and administrators. Second, sport management students create and consider the remarks of others when creating a mission statement. The combination of studying real-world mission statements coupled with the process of developing specific action statements within a mission statement for an institution is enriching and educational.

Activity IV: Schedule Development

The season selected for the scheduling section of the activity—either fall, winter, or spring—can be the choice of the professor. Sport management educators should avoid using the current year academic calendar while incorporating this activity. Athletic schedules are planned months and years in advance. The class activity should also use upcoming year calendars for planning purposes. Students are directed to develop sport schedules of three college-level teams in one season of play.

Directions to Students

Professors can create a lecture based on the need for effective leadership and planning in intercollegiate athletics. The parameters for the start of the season and end of the season must be clarified before the scheduling process. For the fall season the professor, after discussing preseason issues (planning, housing, scrimmages, NCAA rules, institutional restrictions), should select a start date for the entire class to use.

In addition, the class should be given the start date for the regular season (opening day for all teams, for example, Saturday, September 6) and final day of regular season play (for example, Saturday, November 1). The professor can then indicate when the playoffs should end and when the conference champion needs to be crowned to prepare for the NCAA

Women's Soccer Fall Schedule

Date	Opponent	Location	Time
9/2	vs. Babson		7 PM
9/6	at Amherst	Amherst, MA	11 AM
9/12	at Williams	Williams, MA	3 PM
9/15	vs. UMass Boston		7 PM
9/20	at Colby	Waterville, ME	11 AM
9/25	vs. Roger Williams		7 PM
9/29	at St. Anslem	Manchester, NH	7 PM
10/2	vs. Holy Cross		7 PM
10/6	at Wentworth	Boston, MA	7 PM
10/10	at Wheaton	Norton, MA	3 PM
10/13	vs. Roger Williams		7 PM
10/17	at Brandeis	Waltham, MA	3 PM
10/21	vs. Curry		7 PM
10/25	at Eastern Nazarene	Quincy, MA	11 AM
10/28	vs. Rivier		7 PM
11/1	vs. Salem State		11 AM
11/5	vs. Endrcott		7 PM
11/8	at Salve Regina	Newport, RI	11 AM

Tournament in each of the sports. Within the course structure the class can discuss playoff policies and procedures, the advantages and disadvantages of including all conference members in playoff games, the purpose of automatic bids or qualifications into the NCAA tournament, budgeting, transportation, lodging, and meal preparation and planning for playoffs. Students use full-page calendars from August to November to begin the scheduling process in class; within the designated student conferences discussions center on scheduling procedures, and then conferences can create playoff schedule, policies, and procedures.

Scheduling Procedures

Each student schedules two games for each sport between all conference members. If there are six conferences members the total number of conference games for women's soccer is 10. Students then schedule seven nonconference games for each sport. Two preseason competitions/scrimmages are scheduled for each team. According to the NCAA only one date of competition is used for all playoff games, including conference

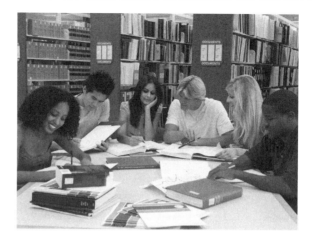

play and NCAA playoffs. The total number of regular season games totals 17, with two scrimmages and one date for postseason play, for a total of 20 dates of competition.

Teaching Tip
Sport management educators can discuss how planning effectively for teams is important for a successful sport season. Professors can discuss the benefits of starting conference play after a few nonconference games have been scheduled.

Teaching Tip
Professors should ensure all students in the class are scheduling the same amount of games. If a conference is smaller or larger than six members, the easiest adjustment is to decrease or increase the number of nonconference games played.

Teaching Tip
Scheduling for preseason scrimmages: Students should be advised not to schedule preseason competitions with conference opponents. A discussion can develop as to the rationale for avoiding scrimmages with any future regular season opponents.

Scheduling Discussions
For students to gain a true understanding of the scheduling process for intercollegiate athletics, professors can provide guidance throughout

the process. Professors can have students start to schedule and then find teachable moments to stop the in-class scheduling work and use examples to help direct students.

Teachable Moments

Each course we teach may contain interesting and intriguing sport management topics. What sets the course apart from others is the pedagogic tools sport management educators incorporate within the class to create dynamic learning environments. This semester-long activity can be the vehicle to enhance student learning through the various stages of the project.

After students have an understanding of the parameters of the scheduling process, such as the number of games and conference members, the scheduling process can begin. Students should have a portion of class time to start their work scheduling with other course mates. During the designated class time the professor initiates the process by having students use their full-page calendar to work on their scheduling tasks. Allow students to meet with course mates and devise agreements with others in the class. After 10 minutes the sport management professor can stop and ask students to explain their status of scheduling games.

Issues

Students may remain in their conference group to devise their conference schedule first. For those who do not, this is a beneficial time to explore the rationale for setting up the conference schedule before all other contests. The primary reason for this is that the conference schedule is more important than all other games. Students schedule conference games early in the season instead of considering playing nonconference contests for the teams to build a more cohesive unit and be better prepared for the all important conference matchups.

Students may schedule multiple games in a row. Professors can address this issue now or wait for the schedules to be submitted. A discussion can explore the rationale for playing games in a method using a rotation of Tuesday–Thursday–Saturday contests one week followed by Wednesday–Saturday contests in the following weeks. The purpose for the combinations is that students traveling to away contests are not faced with missing class time. Alternating the rotation of games takes into consideration academic schedules and in some cases may avoid conflicts between athletics and academics.

Start times of games also draw a great deal of discourse when considering the scheduling process. Sport management professors can ask students when the best time to start games would be. The discussion of start times can lead to a wide array of issues faced by student-athletes when balancing and juggling the rigor of academics with the physical and mental demands of collegiate athletics. Students need to take into consideration start times for evening/night games. Once students complete a draft of their schedule, professors can spend time commenting on start times. As an athletic administrator students need to consider a 7:30 PM start time for an away game during the week that is 4 hours away from campus. Students must also understand the impact of multiple late start times for one team over the course of the season. In some instances students may also schedule back-to-back games during the week. Best practices in scheduling suggest avoiding back-to-back games whenever possible for the health and benefit of the teams. In some cases back-to-back Saturday and Sunday games are common practice for athletic conferences. Professors can decide if weekend games played back to back are acceptable for this project.

Discussion Points in Class

Two elements stressed in the class are to promote the thinking that students should represent themselves like athletic administrators at all times (when submitting assigned work or through verbal/written expression) and at the same time become gender-neutral thinkers when sharing perspectives and making decisions. Setting gender-neutral attitudes creates safe boundaries for all students, especially in a course where sensitive topics such as gender equity, Title IX, and major versus minor sports are examined. The following discussion points allow sport management professors to assess the thought process and decision-making capacities of students in a group setting:

- Describe how your athletic departments will ensure a culture of gender fairness.
- Describe your opening talk to student-athletes regarding the issues of hazing.
- What questions would you ask a potential candidate for the assistant athletic director position at your institution?
- Prepare a statement to the Board of Trustees to justify the addition of a new stadium for your fall teams (women's soccer and men's soccer only).

Scheduling Assignments

The following assignments are to be completed by students and collected 2 weeks after start of scheduling.

1. *Conference playoff policy.* The written policy and conference tournament should be approved by the professor early in the semester to ensure proper scheduling, time between games, and inclusion of all conference

members in playoffs. The policy should include number of teams included in conference playoff tournament, the conference bracket set-up once teams are seeded, the policy for seeding teams, and the location and time of games.

Teaching Tip

Professors can take time to discuss how teams are seeded from numbers 1 to 6 for example. The conferences can decide to use winning percentage (number of wins divided by the number of total games played or number of wins plus .5 [tie/draw] divided by number of total games played) or a point system (3 points for a win, 1 point for a tie/draw, 0 points for loss). The professor can illustrate the differences and perspectives for using each of these scoring systems. Once the games are played later in the semester, students calculate their winning percentage or points earned for each sport and for conference play, nonconference play, and total games played (including all regular season games, conference and nonconference). Students may ask if scrimmages/preseason games are included in the scoring system, which they are not. In fact, professors can discuss the issues of even web posting of scores and results from a scrimmage, which in essence is a friendly match to fine-tune the team for the regular season.

Teaching Tip

One of the most important aspects of policy development is to have steps in place to resolve an issue. Many times teams within a conference have identical conference records. To accurately place teams in the correct standings, a tiebreak procedure must be constructed. Students can be directed to find procedures currently used by college athletic conferences to provide a perspective on the issue.

There are some simple methods for organizing a tiebreak (each professor and class can decide the best method to be incorporated) if the conference record for two or more teams is identical:

a. Determine conference record: use the agreed on scoring system (winning percentage or points). The scoring system cannot change just to decide a tiebreak.

b. Determine the record against higher seeded teams in the conference. The team with the best record against the common higher seeded team gets to move ahead. In the case of multiple teams in a tiebreak situation continue to place teams based on the second and third best records against higher seeded teams. If the teams are still tied, then move to step c.

    c. Determine record against common opponent. The team with the best record against the common opponent gets to move ahead. In the case of multiple teams in a tiebreak situation continue to place teams based on the second and third best records against higher seeded teams. If the teams are still tied, then move to step d.

    d. Determine the amount of goals scored against your team in conference play and with common and nonconference opponents.

    e. If a tie continues after steps a–d, a simple rule of thumb is to use a coin toss to determine the seeding.

Teaching Tip

Professors can discuss the rationale for using goals against statistics versus goals scored (goals for). In some cases when the tiebreak uses goals scored, teams may feel the need to "run up" the score of the game, and athletic teams may see some very lopsided results. When instituting goals against, this statistic focuses on the amount of goals opponents scored while playing a team. To stay consistent when determining the tiebreaker, conference should rely on goals against for conference play; then if a tie persists the conference can look at goals against for common nonconference opponents.

    2. *Draft of schedule 3 to 4 weeks into the semester.* Students need to be diligent in their working meetings with course mates before class, being active during designated class time, and using the course management system to schedule games. Once the draft is collected, the professor can assess the progress of each student.

Teaching Tip

Here are some specific items to look for:

- What did the student prioritize in terms of games scheduled? Was the focus on scrimmages, nonconference games, and conference games?
- Has the student plotted all necessary start dates and dates of importance on the calendar as a reference when completing the scheduling tasks? For example, student should have plotted on their calendars the preseason start date, first day of class, end of regular season date, conference playoffs and pairings, end of conference tournament play, and start of NCAA tournament.
- The proper spacing between games: Did the students create a system of scheduling following a Tuesday–Thursday–Saturday and Wednesday–Saturday rotation?

- ○ Priority to Saturday games: Most fall athletic teams play games on Saturday. The rationale for Saturday contests is that first student-athletes do not miss class time, the campus can support and watch the games, and parents/friends are free and available to view games on the weekend.
- Were start times of games included?
- Were back-to-back games used?
- Were the following proper format and codes used in the schedule?
  MS (H) 4 PM Gentile State College
  WS (A) 7 PM Gentile State College
  FH (H) 4 PM Gentile State College
- Is there a balance between number of home and away contests?
- Are class absences required for each athletic contest (start times)?
- Have dates for conference playoffs and NCAA tournament been included?
- Are facilities available on a specific date and time?

Activity V: Travel Needs

One aspect of organizing athletic schedules is to determine distance to travel to away contests, mode of transportation, lodging, and meal costs and plans. To get a true sense of the process, students develop a travel grid for conference games. The sport management professor can select to have students create travel grids (**Figure 3.1**) for all away contests or just for conference opponents.

Students use popular travel websites to determine actual mileage and travel time for athletic teams traveling from campus to campus. A discussion can develop based on planning for away travel, including how much time each team/coach may require for pregame preparations. In regards to meal preparation and athletic contests, it is important for future athletic

Figure 3.1 Sample Travel Grid

	Gentile State	University of Quinn	Laine College
Gentile State		100 miles 2.5 hrs	50 miles 1 hr
University of Quinn	100 miles 2.5 hrs		180 miles 3 hrs
Laine College	50 miles 1 hr	180 miles 3 hrs	

administrators to be concerned about the nutritional health of student-athletes. The sport management professor may lead a lecture regarding using meal money (funding provided by the athletic department) or "brown bag" meals provided by the campus dining hall. Students who are currently athletes may argue for meal money for each away trip. The sport management professor can begin to discuss the budgetary procedures for athletic departments along with the need for policies and procedures to be carefully structured when dealing with institutional dollars. A policy for meal plans for away contests may state the following: "Each athletic team shall have three away contests in which meals will be funded by the athletic department." Another policy may indicate that no team shall use more than three "brown bag" meals on consecutive away contests. Typical allocation of funding for each student-athlete for away contests is $5 for breakfast, $8 for lunch, and $10 for dinner. In addition, the sport management professor can also discuss the importance of each coach completing and submitting an expense report at the end of the away trip to provide a check and balance system to account for all monies spent.

For the purposes of this activity the sport management professor is at liberty to decide whether or not to include one weekend in which teams will be lodging at a hotel. The format of discussion is similar to that required for the meal-planning process. Students can research hotel costs and availability if lodging is an option for the team(s). The activity may demonstrate how difficult in may be to find lodging in a "popular tourist" area during scheduled games or even during an opponent's Family or Homecoming Weekend.

Activity VI: Contract Signing

Creating a "contract signing activity" is a checks and balance system to ensure students have scheduled the correct amount of contests with other students in class, to determine if the dates and times correspond, and if students did not over- or under-schedule athletic contests. To get a taste of the scheduling process students create their own contract with institution name and logo and conference logo.

Contents of an athletic contract, which is a memorandum of understanding, include the date, time, sport, location of the contest, and any special provisions (for example, Alumni Weekend). The contract is signed by both representatives of the athletic institutions.

To create a system of cross-checking that students have scheduled the correct amount of contests and contests with the "correct" course mate(s), students include all signed copies of the contracts. Sport management professors can organize the method of contract signing in several fashions. Students should understand the process and purpose of contract signing. First, contracts are in fact binding agreements when signed by authorized college personnel. Second, contracts are used to handle any disputes between institutions regarding field, time, and date of contest. Third, the process is a confirmation of the scheduled games for the upcoming seasons.

Activity VII: Contest Management

Budgeting

Students develop complete budgets for the cost associated with operating home contests. In addition, students develop budgets for the travel and meal costs associated with away contests. Students are required to use Excel spreadsheets for budget construction and submission.

Home Game Cost Application

Sport management professors can set the number of personnel to be hired, the costs for specific items, and salary structure so that all students are working with same monetary figures. The following costs can be explored through a designated class lecture and discussion:

- *Work study staff:* Full-time staff member salaries do not need to be included in the calculations for home game costs. Work study students can be hired for the following areas: ball retrieval people (two work study students), scoreboard operator (one student), and concession stand workers (two work study students). Professors can review the amount of time (hours) each person will be expected to work for a home contest. Consideration must be given to double headers planned for a specific date along with any provisions for overtime games. Sport management professors can set the work study wage and review the formula for calculating the cost for all work study students used for the event(s).
- *Officials:* Sport management professors can lead discussions relating to the cost and number of officials used for fall, winter, and spring sport teams. For the purposes of this exercise students create budgets for fall sport teams only. Students calculate the season costs for the hiring of officials for men's soccer, women's soccer, and women's field hockey. The assumption is one center official for men's and women's soccer games (cost, $120 dollars), two assistant referees for men's and women's soccer (cost, $100 per official), and two officials for field hockey (cost, $100 per official).

Away Game Cost Application

Determining the costs associated with away games requires more planning and information. Students now refer to their created schedules to calculate and determine the actual costs for managing the team budgets for away contests. The following costs can be explored through a designated class lecture and discussion:

- *Transportation:* Sport management professors can predetermine what modes of transportation are acceptable for team travel. Each student uses the same cost for the use of vans ($100 per van) or the use of a chartered bus ($300).
- *Meals:* A clear policy must be created to determine the distribution of meal funds or the use of dining hall services for team meals for away contests. Students use the created game times to determine which meals will be consumed by teams on the road.
- *Lodging:* Sport management professors can decide if any lodging is necessary for this section of the project. If lodging is used, students should use a set figure for rooms needed for the team and the cost per room. Sport management professors can preset these figures so that all students are working with the same figures.

Teaching Tip

Sport management professors can take advantage of academic technology by scheduling a few blocks of class time in a college computer room so students can get exposed to using a practical tool for creating schedules and budgets. The in-class Excel labs require that each student bring his or her initial budget requests to class to assist in the data manipulation and spreadsheet development.

Homecoming Weekend and Campus Special Events

One method to simulate the chore of athletic scheduling is to plan for and plan around special campus events and Homecoming/Family/Alumni Weekends. Sport management faculty members can add a special campus event or even a water main break during the scheduling process. Students must then reschedule athletic contests. This process allows students to communicate with their peers, negotiate with course mates, and represent the interests of their campuses. In addition, all fall sport teams must also be concerned with Homecoming Weekend, which typically falls during the last weekend of September through October. Using a class-generated memo the sport management professor, who is the acting athletic director, sends an internal memo to each student. The memo states that all fall teams are required by the Office of the President to play a home game on Homecoming Weekend. The sport management professor randomly assigns the Homecoming date to each student. The date can be selected at the same time the sport management professor is reviewing the draft of the fall calendar created by the student. The sport management professor can decide to select a date that is not currently filled, a date when all teams are playing away contests, or a date when one of the three teams are slated to play at home.

Activity VIII: Playing the Games

One of the greatest joys of this project is seeing the process through to the end. Students are able to play out their schedules and playoffs in the "roll off." Each student uses one die to roll their score. The class must have ground rules for the "roll off." Some simple guidelines include rolling date by date according to the created schedule (scrimmages do not have to be played for this activity), keeping track of scores (students may need to calculate goals scored and goals against), recording all game results, and playing overtime if there is a tie/draw according to the rules set by the NCAA. For women's soccer as an example, if the game is tied after one roll, students roll again for overtime; if it is still tied, they roll one more time (this would simulate the shoot out). Checking the NCAA for the rules each semester is helpful because overtime regulations may be revised from season to season and sport to sport.

It is also important that students learn the proper mechanisms for reporting the scores/results of the games played. The acceptable method is as follows:

- W 1–0: Team won one goal to no goals
- L 0–1: Team lost no goals to one goal
- T 0–0 (OT): Teams tied zero to zero in one overtime period
- T 1–1 (2OT): Teams tied one to one in two overtime periods
- W 2–1 (2OT): Team won two goals to one goal in two overtime periods
- L 1–2 (2OT): Team lost one goal to two goals in two overtime periods.

After all regular season games have been played and are accurately reported, conference members meet again in their groups to determine the conference playoff seedings (**Figure 3.2**). This process takes some time because

Figure 3.2 Tournament Bracket

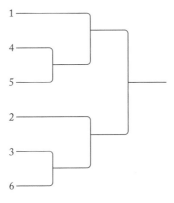

students need to document their wins and losses for all conference games and present records for all games played. Once the seedings are developed and set, the conference members create playoff pairings and brackets. The conference playoff games are then played until a conference winner in each sport is crowned.

Once the conference championships have concluded, all conference winners are then seeded for the 1-day NCAA championship tournament. The championship tournament brackets are then created based on winning percentage or points earned according to the policy created within the class. Once the pairings are set, students roll off to determine the overall class winner in each sport. This is a terrific concluding activity after a time-consuming, thought-provoking, and challenging semester-long project.

Activity IX: State of Athletics

After all schedules have been created and all season games played, students now have the opportunity to reflect on the year and present their findings to the Board of Trustees at their institution. The written "State of Athletics" report can take a variety of forms according to the creativity of the individual student. Each student must, however, recap the season providing details of regular season records, conference records and playoff results, and overall team records. Students can reflect on the year, stressing the positive factors and the benefits of intercollegiate athletic competitions, along with any changes they as athletic administrators may make to provide a more comprehensive and successful athletic program on and off the playing surfaces.

Activity X: Off-Season Tournament Development

Another aspect of the process is to allow students to prepare for the ever popular off-season schedules of athletic teams at all levels. Within this course activity students select a weekend date (Saturday or Sunday) for one of their fall teams to host a spring tournament. The tournament must be advertised to course mates, and students are required to secure a minimum of five teams for the play day. For the other two fall sports, students participate in two play days hosted by another institution.

Components of the activity are as follows:

- Develop a one-page handout to promote the event.
- Set a fee for institutions to pay for the event.
- Create the play day schedule, with a minimum number of guaranteed games or brackets.
- Provide incentives if necessary to attract teams to event.
- Participate in two play days for other non-hosting team.
- Play the event using the roll off.
- Submit complete bracket and end of tournament recap.

Teaching Tip

For an online activity, students can set up a blog or web page for their tournament and solicit course mates to participate in their event.

Activity XI: Hiring Plan

Sport management professors can spend time reviewing the wide variety of athletic department positions and job titles in intercollegiate athletics (**Figure 3.3**). Students can navigate sites such as NCAA.org to research job opportunities and position openings in intercollegiate athletics across the country. For this activity students create a list of potential personnel to be hired. Students include job title, some key components of the position, required educational background, and suggested salary. The activity lends itself to a larger discussion of job description development and entry- and advanced-level salaries for professionals in athletic administrations. Students can also review the *NCAA News*, to which most athletic departments subscribe, for job postings and positions to help formulate a hiring plan for their institution.

Activity XII: Written Institutional Policies and Procedures

To provide students with the ground work to assist in building their own fundamental framework of decision making, sport management professors

Figure 3.3 Athletic Department Flow Chart

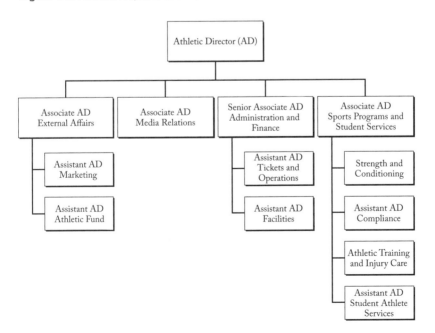

can assign a project in which students research common policy and procedures for athletic departments and the develop their own comprehensive document. Students systematically determine what guidelines and regulations they need to create to run an efficient athletic department.

Sport management students create a policy and procedure manual for their uniquely created institution. The comprehensive document should serve to guide the athletic department staff and coaches on the operating procedures of the department. Policy is developed for the following sections.

Part I: Marketing the Institution

Students create an athletics recruiting guide to assist the Admissions Office with the recruitment of student-athletes. The material can be submitted in booklet format, including logo development and graphics to assist in communicating the positive attributes of the institution. The athletic guide is a marketing publication to recruit student-athletes and to provide information regarding academic program offerings and athletic opportunities at the institution. The following items should be included:
- Location and characteristics of the institution
- Characteristics of student-athletes (who are they, where do they reside, average standardized test scores, average grade point average)
- Athletic facilities (indoor and outdoor features)
- Institutional philosophy (academic, athletic, team/sport objectives and goals)
- Conference affiliation (list of conference members)

Part II: Staff Policies and Procedures

The contents developed for this section serve to guide the staff of the athletic department. Students should understand that if the staff person in athletics has a question regarding any of the included areas, they can read the written policy and have all the requisite information to guide them appropriately. In addition to written policies, students develop forms that are associated with the specific policy and procedure that are used for the operation of the athletic department. Items to include are as follows:
- *An overview of the fiscal management and philosophy of the athletic department:* This section may also include college-wide procedures as well. Students provide clear and concise details on purchasing, check requests, and purchase requisitions. Forms can be used to appropriately direct the reader.
- *Hiring plan (athletic personnel):* Students create a list of essential personnel for the athletic department including job descriptions for each. The purpose of the exercise is to allow students to

think through the hiring process for their newly created institution. In addition, students get an understanding of the hierarchy that will be developed for their athletic department. Students are directed to create one general job description for all coaches and to simply list all sport coaches in the department. Students also create a visual flow chart to demonstrate the importance of clear reporting lines and to develop an accountable paper trail for their institution. Along with job descriptions, students create job titles for each of the athletic department staff members.

- *Student athletic eligibility and academic requirements:* Within this section students can research similar athletic institutions to develop an academic policy for student-athlete eligibility for athletic participation. Students should be able to create a standard for minimum number of course credits and minimum grade point average for athletic participation eligibility. In addition, students create a plan to assist in the monitoring of student-athletes and a policy for ineligible student-athletes.
- *Specific athletic department program policies:*
  - *Preseason (fall, winter, and spring sports):* Students develop the procedure for inviting student-athletes to attend preseason along with the number of scrimmages for each team.
  - *Scheduling:* For this section students must ensure the reader understands the scheduling process, the staff person responsible and accountable for the schedule, the role of the head coach in the process, the minimum and maximum number of games per sport (fall, winter, spring), and pertinent conference scheduling information.
  - *Team size:* To create equity across all programs, students are guided to list the maximum number of team members (excluding coaches) for each sport offered at the institution. In addition, students can list the number of student-athletes who travel to away contests if it is different from the stated roster size.
  - *Scouting:* An overall policy for all coaches can be listed for scouting opponents. The assumption is that no tape exchanges currently occur for conference members. The policy should explain the role of the head coach and the travel reimbursement (if any) for travel to watch and evaluate upcoming opponents.
  - *Recruitment:* The policy should include on-campus visitation of eligible student-athletes, overnight visitation procedures and acceptable weeknight dates, and classroom observation information.

- *Behavioral guidelines for student-athletes:* This section provides detailed outlines for any behavioral policies for the athletic department at the college or university. Students develop policies for substance abuse, discrimination, harassment, and hazing. The policy can be written for athletic department personnel and for student-athletes. Some athletic departments may develop their own student-athlete handbook, and students in the course should understand the policies for this activity are read by departmental staff and must be followed by the athletic department staff.

Activity XIII: Website Development

Collegiate athletics has turned the corner on the use of technology to showcase their athletic teams, report results, advertise for sponsors, and be a source of information for the community. Students in any sport management course can be guided to create a free website using some of the Internet host sites. Some sites include pbwiki.com, geocities.com, and weebly.com.

For this activity students are required to create their own individual website for their created institution. In addition, students are asked to create a conference website to work together in the conference setting. The conference website must have links and interaction with all conference members. Students present their conference and institutional website to the class. The best conference website as voted by the class can earn extra credit as an incentive.

....

Teaching Tip

Another method to get students to take pride and ownership while creating their website is to have each student post their work on the course website. Students will take extra care when their peers can view their work. In addition, students can learn from the work of others and may reach out for help and assistance.

Activity XIV: Professional Presentation

At the conclusion of the semester-long project, students have 5 to 8 minutes to address the class. Students select the athletic issue they wish to address and to whom they are speaking. Example of issue or topics can be

- Orientation for new coaches
- Welcome address and information for preseason players and families
- Open house event addressing student-athletes and families
- Application to join a new athletic conference

Students are guided to use the allocated time to showcase their institution using the information and assignments created throughout the semester including team records and conference standings. Overall, students are required to prepare a professional and engaging presentation that provides information and guidance.

Questions to Consider

- Which types of projects can you embed into your courses that build on prior knowledge and are comprehensive in nature?
- What important issues could you include in this type of course that is reflective of current challenges athletic administrators must resolve?
- How can you foster and nurture an environment of gender neutrality in courses that deal with athletic programs and equity in sport?

4

Teaching Activities: Financial Management

The umbrella topic of financial management most likely is addressed in a number of courses throughout a typical 4-year program of study in sport management. The activities included in this financial management chapter can be used in a variety of courses, such as Introduction to Sport Management, Management of Sport Organization, Administration of Sport, and Sport Finance and Economics. Depending on the course level sport management educators who teach financial management can sequentially add pieces to the financial management topic(s) addressed in their courses. When multiple faculty members instruct courses that include budget or financial management, it may be beneficial for all professors to discuss which types of activities they will incorporate in their teaching and course materials to avoid duplication of assignments and/or projects.

This chapter explores the following teaching activities in financial management:

- Budget creation
- Financial management decision making
- Stock market awareness
- Business plan creation and analysis
- Professional sport leagues and financial challenges

Organization of Lecture and Class Discourse

Sport management educators can lead an active discussion relating to the issues affecting sport management and athletic administration from a financial perspective. To engage the class professors can start to define revenue and revenue streams (generation) for three types of sport management industries: health fitness club, college athletic department (Division I), and professional sport franchise. Students can join a group and discuss common revenue sources common for these three sport entities.

Such issues in health fitness club are memberships, merchandise, class fees, and health food purchases. For a Division I college athletic department students may consider ticket sales, stadium revenue (rental), merchandise, concessions, media guide sales, and sponsorships. For a professional sport franchise revenue sources can consist of media agreements, ticket sales, merchandise, sponsorship, league profit sharing, hospitality, and parking fees.

After that exercise the discussion can move into practical decision making in an ever-changing financial environment. At this juncture sport management professors can review the components of a situational analysis for sport businesses. Students can be exposed to the various factors and components that assist sport managers in making financial and management decisions. One component of the situational analysis includes monitoring the internal and external environments of a sport entity. Internal environmental factors are concentrated in the components a sport manager can control. Sport management professors can pose the question to students by asking to list factors under the control of a fitness manager or retail sporting goods manager. For the most part fitness managers can control for the marketing of membership services, employing staffing and training, the hours of operation, and the types of services offered. On the external environment side students must understand there are numerous and inevitable factors in the workplace that we cannot predict with certainty. To minimize risk sport management must be able to forecast and anticipate changes in the marketplace. Some of the external factors we cannot predict with accuracy are social trends and behaviors, economic hardships, technological advances, competitor advances in the marketplace, and changes in the political or legislative sectors that impact sport business.

Class Discussion

Sport management professors can examine rising gas prices as an example of adapting based on changes in the external environment. Athletic programs that must transport teams throughout the year from one campus to the next must find cost-saving mechanisms to provide a quality athletic experience to student-athletes and supporters. Students can be asked to brainstorm ideas to fulfill the athletic schedule while maintaining the budget line.

From the professional sport perspective, with an economy under financial constraints how can professional sport teams compete for the "entertainment dollar" or the discretionary income of sport consumers? In addition, students can suggest and list new types of revenue streams or methods of generating revenue that teams have not yet considered in their current marketplace.

"Doing more with less" seems to be the directive that athletic administrators operate under in current times. Students are prompted to outline some of the struggles athletic administrators encounter when operating their fiscal budgets. In addition, the class can offer their own experiences (personal and professional) with fiscal management or budget management. Based on the progression of the discussion, sport management professors can incorporate common definitions of the following terms: budget, budgeting, accounting, finance, types of budgets, operating budgets, capital budgets, balance sheet, income statement, and capital equipment. These concepts can be integrated into subsequent assignments and serve to clarify budget terminology for students.

In addition, students need to comprehend the differences in the fiscal year for educational institutions versus the corporate setting. Students can be exposed to the two types of fiscal year systems (the 12-month period when the sport entity operates the budget) used by athletic departments (July 1 to June 30) and public sport entities (January 1 to December 31). Other terminology to be clarified for and by students includes expenses, supplies, and the variations in systems of budgeting in both the educational and corporate settings.

Activity I: Interview With a Financial Manager in Sports

Students in a first-year sport management course may have little to no experience with financial management or budgeting. For students to get insight into the topic of sport finance, instructors can require students to spend time learning about budgets through face-to-face or phone interviews with a sport manager. Often, students complete an internship during their first year or study. In many internship settings students are exposed to budgetary and financial issues. It is therefore important that students have, at a minimum, a surface level understanding of financial management. One opportunity to learn more about the budgeting process is to interview a professional within the industry who manages budgets and handles financial decision making on a daily basis.

Teaching Tip

To avoid duplications in the interview selections, students must post their person of interest in the designated forum within a course website. Students understand that once a person is selected they must use a second candidate for the assignment.

Over a number of years of conducting this assignment, it has become clear that students benefit from a guide of questions to ask finance professionals. The questions also create a level of consistency throughout the class. Students are able to compare and differentiate between their findings and the information provided by course mates.

Sample Interview Format and Questions

1. Interview one sport manager who is in charge of a budget (e.g., fitness club manager, sports camp director, athletic director, professional sports financial executive, intramural director).
2. From the interview, determine who is responsible for the budgeting process and what policies are associated with budgetary decision making within that organization.
3. How often is the budget revised, and what type of input does the budget manager collect from department heads within the organization?
4. Do all employees have access to budget information? Why or why not?
5. How are budget figures derived from year to year, sport to sport, or season to season?
6. What does the budget/financial manager believe are the three most important facets associated with the budget process, and how do they communicate these tenets to others in the organization?
7. Ultimately, who in the organization must be accountable for the budgeting process?

Students write and submit a report of their findings. The report can be an analysis of their findings and the most intriguing information collected through the interview process. Students are encouraged to ask follow-up questions and have a preset number of content-related questions they would like to ask before the interview. Professors can review the list of questions students will be using for the project, or students can discuss their list with one or two other course mates during class time or through an online discussion forum.

....

Teaching Tip

Be sure students understand that an interview must occur either face to face or over the telephone. Often, students e-mail the questions and the interviewee e-mails the responses. This prevents students from participating in a rich learning environment of public speaking. Correspondence interviewing prohibits students from learning in real time, students cannot ask follow-up questions, and the personal connection with the financial expert is minimized.

_____

Activity II: Budget Creation and Decision-Making Simulation

Using financial management as the topic for discussion, students are asked to create two start-up budgets for two college sports teams.

Step I: Instructors can ask students to determine equipment, supplies, and salaries needed for the entire academic year. In addition, reference pages are required to support the listed dollar amounts. To get a well-represented pool of male and female sports, instructors can assign teams or place limitations on the use of one team sport and one individual sport.

Step II: Once the students complete the budgets, they are asked to share their work with one other student in the class. If the course is delivered online, students can share files to complete the activity. For a traditional face-to-face course students can sit next to each other and spend time reviewing each other's work. Students are then asked to use a critical eye and to indicate what budget items or necessary information is missing from their partner's work. Students must indicate if items such as jersey color, short size, numbering, vendor information, item description, cost, and date needed were overlooked by their partner.

Step III: In this stage students act as the athletic director, and with the budget total submitted for the teams they must direct their partner to cut the budgets by 10%. Students have an opportunity to exercise their negotiating skills, and those who are facing budget cuts learn to come up with creative ways to salvage their budgets for their sport teams. The activity is a learning experience, whereby students get to wear two different hats in the financial decision making in the budget process.

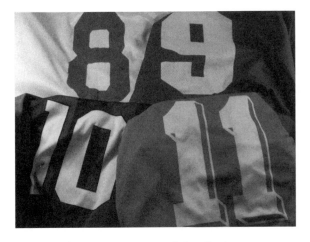

Activity III: Budget Creation and Analysis

Students are asked to create three types of budgets. The budget scenario can take any form: a week-long summer camp, a fundraising event, a fitness club renovation, or a sport apparel start-up company. Students use the information from the lectures, readings, and reference materials to complete and create these athletic budgets. By using electronic spreadsheets students are required to detail the items for inclusion for the budgets. Sport management educators can use a computer-based tutorial to explain the necessary details of budget construction. Incorporating software into this activity allows students to experience technology in the classroom.

Including written analysis and a rationale for the budgetary information allows sport management educators to assess student's acquisition of knowledge in creating budgets. Students spend time thinking through the essential components of a budget.

Content for Budget and Analysis

- *Policy:* Professors can provide information as to the role of policy and decision maker on the amount of funding for a particular department or individual event(s).
- *Philosophy:* At the heart of budget development is the philosophy sport managers adopt as budget administrators. A portion of the discussion on financial management centers on the types of administrators and how personal and professional management styles and philosophy play a role in the type of financial leader one may become.
- *Systems approach:* Sport management professors can discuss the interconnectedness of departments and/or athletic teams as it relates to budgeting. Students at this level can get an understanding that all departments/teams may be competing for the same pool of

funds. The system of budgeting the sport manager or athletic director adopts dictates the type of funding received.

- *Equity:* As all departments and teams compete for the various dollar amounts, sport administrators must be sure to make fair decisions in regards to the needs of all programs. From an athletic perspective, sport management educators can devote time and share information regarding gender equity in athletics. Gender fairness and equity applies to the fundamental decisions made by athletic administrators.

- *Bottom line:* Sport management students must also be sure to understand the significance and impact of their decisions. Sport management students need to be accountable for adhering to that bottom line, especially when it comes to financial management in the sport business setting.

Once the budgets are complete, students are asked to trade their budgets with one other student in the class to get feedback from someone other than the sport management professor. Students then have an opportunity to discuss the contents of the budget, any missing items, issues with miscalculations, issues with missed cost applications, and overall review of the contents of the created budgets. Students are expected to bring their calculators to adequately review and assess the budgets.

Activity IV: Stock Market Awareness

Information relating to the stock market is more available to our students than ever before. Popular television programs that cover "current and hot" financial topics and stories are viewed by college age students. The following is a simple method to teach about the stock market. As an example, students

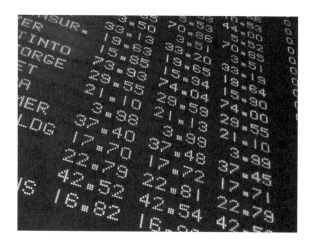

are asked to log onto Yahoo.com, select finance, and type in Under Armour (or any sport organization that is publicly traded). Sport management educators can select more than one sport-related company for use in this activity. Students review the company financials and stock performance over a designated time period. Instructors through this activity encourage students to discuss the company, its history, and what the financial statements tell the general public about the company.

Teaching Tip

This can be completed online (within the course website). Students post their analysis of the designated company with the understanding they cannot duplicate the information provided by others. Students can forecast the future offerings of the company.

Follow-Up: In the Current Marketplace

Students also can be asked to find a current article that discusses the financial outlook of the designated company and to share their findings with the class.

Teaching Tip

This activity can be incorporated with a course website for traditional face-to-face courses. For online courses this material can be placed in a forum or discussion board. In either scenario students will link the reference material or article, post a summary of the article, and ask two follow-up questions to the group. Students are then responsible for responding to each other's work and analysis. For larger classes instructors may ask that students respond to only three others or designate smaller work groups for the responses.

Activity V: Stock Ownership

The following activity can be incorporated in upper level sport management/finance courses. Students conduct a search of four sport-related companies that offer publicly traded stocks. The list can include companies that sponsor sporting events or manufacture sport products and services. Students start with four companies before a final company is selected using a lottery system. Students randomly select a card with a number. The student with the lowest number selects his or her primary choice for the assignment, and the process continues until all students have a company to research.

Teaching Tip

The lottery system eliminates duplication of companies. In addition, if one student's list has been exhausted through the process, other students have three other choice companies they can share with course mates.

Teaching Tip

For online courses, to avoid duplication students can be randomly assigned a selection order by the instructor, or a first-post, first-pick process can be used through a designated forum or discussion board.

Sport Company Stock Analysis Project

To start the process of buying stock, students are given $10,000 of classroom currency. Instructors can now use the formulas presented in **Box 4.1** to determine the amount of stock owned by each student. Students can be directed to use common stock calculations for their assignments.

BOX 4.1 Stock Calculations

To determine the number of shares purchased with an original investment:

Original investment ÷ stock price = number of shares

To determine current value of the purchased stock:

Number of shares owned × closing price = current value

To determine profit or loss:

Current value − original investment = profit or loss

(Students must understand that a stock owner only loses or gains once the stock is sold.)

Over a designated time period students monitor the progress of their stock. Throughout this time instructors can check in on the progress of the companies. Students may find that a stock has split. This is a perfect occasion to teach the concepts of a stock split.

Stock Split

At times companies make a decision to split the current stock. The most common type of split is 2 for 1. The stock price at this point is cut in half and the amount of shares owned is doubled. There are multiple reasons why companies may split stocks. One reason is that the stock price may be too high for the intended market and therefore out of reach or unattractive to the general public. To appeal more to the general target groups, companies perform a stock split.

Stock Performance Presentation

Students begin to take ownership of this activity. You may experience students bragging about how well their stock is performing, whereas others make little gains or big losses. The experience allows students to analyze one company and to feel connected to the process because they have classroom currency committed to the activity.

At the conclusion of the project students can present the information they collected from the stock market experience. The following items can be addressed in the presentation:

- *Overview of company:* Company name, any name changes, corporate history, significant historical information, core product and/or product extensions, stock exchange on which the stock is traded, information on corporate headquarters, size and scope of the company, any information regarding parent company, and recent acquisitions and/or mergers are all pertinent information.
- *Financial information:* Students have a time period to investigate and explore the company. Students will find a wide variety of information on popular stock trading websites. Information for the paper/presentation can include income statement analysis, statement of cash flows, balance sheets, and earning reports. In addition, students can share information regarding recent corporate decisions and any major capital expenditures.
- *Current value of the investment:* Students can track the stock performance for a designated time period during the term or semester as decided by the course instructor.
- *Recommendations to the class:* Buy or sell? Students can provide a brief summary including their personal recommendation to invest in the company. Students have the opportunity to review gain/loss over the designated time period. In addition, students try to predict the future of the company based on the research and analysis of current marketplace data and information.

Written Report

Sport management professors, as part of the stock market research, can require students to create a written report of their experience working with one publicly traded company. Instructors can include similar material as required for the presentation or allow students to write a report of their findings from a financial consultation perspective. Students can provide an industry analysis where they analyze the segment of the sport management industry in which the company is involved. Students also explore information regarding past, present, and future trends of the industry. A portion of the research can be an exploration of primary company rivals and competitors. The consultation perspective allows students to synthesize the materials they have collected over the designated time frame, forecast future trends in the marketplace, and make recommendations to potential investors.

Activity VI: Financial Management Group Work

Students in upper level sport management or sport finance courses can get a sense of the financial climate of professional sports leagues. Sport management instructors can assign students to research designated teams in the National Basketball Association, Women's National Basketball Association, National Football League, National Hockey League, Major League Baseball, Women's Professional Soccer, and Major League Soccer, as examples. In addition, sport management educators may also want students to research leagues in Europe, Asia, and Australia. The heart of the research rests with students being able to research and learn about the similarities and differences of two franchises within the league, which includes one large market team and one small market team. The following areas can be included in the portion of the research project:

- Description and selection of teams
- Rationale for selection of small and large market teams for designated league
- Overview and historical background of the team and any special distinctions
- Current ownership and review of past owners (describes the unique background of ownership and its connection to the professional sport)
- Purchase price of franchise and other sale prices
- Current franchise value, as compared to other teams in the same league
- Financial management questions:
  - How the financial climate within the general economy and league specific has changed within the last 3 years
  - The tangible changes these teams have made to adapt to changes in the economy
  - A review of the type of business structure adopted by the league

- ○ Description of the features and uniqueness of league-wide salary regulations and salary caps as well as an analysis of revenue sharing within the league
- Stadium data and information:
  - ○ Collection of information regarding stadium construction
  - ○ Team attendance figures
  - ○ Review of past trends and propose future trends on ticket prices and sales
- Sources of revenue, such as gate receipts (effects of home and away ticket sales), media revenue (deals and agreements with local, national, cable television, web-casting, and radio)
- Stadium revenue, such as ticketing, luxury seating (if appropriate), concessions and merchandise, package deals (hospitality and tickets), souvenir sales
- Costs and expenditures, such as player costs (salary, acquisition costs, signing bonuses, performance bonuses, insurance, and pensions)
- General operating costs, such as rental expenses, administrative payroll

Activity VII: Business Plan Creation and Analysis

Many sport management students may consider starting a new venture within an existing organization or as an entrepreneur. Numerous online tools exist to guide sport management students in understanding the purpose along with the scope of business plan development.

First, students develop a new venture. Each student creates a new company that produces only one product or one service. The goal of the exercise is to allow students to creatively craft an idea for practical use. To track and assess student learning throughout the term or semester, students submit pieces of the project as benchmarkings throughout the term or semester.

Stage I: Idea formulation. This stage includes a company mission statement, goals, objectives, and a description of the product or service. At this stage in the process the sport management professor can provide insightful information to mold the students into the right direction for the activity. Students can be encouraged to investigate a venture they are interested in pursuing for an internship or career.

Stage II: Target market development. It goes without saying that if a new product or service hits the marketplace there needs to be a connection to a core market of consumers. Students research and share the data collected as they prove their product will effectively survive in the competitive marketplace. Students should incorporate current data and research to support their defined core market.

Stage III: Scanning the sport industry environment. Students can understand the limitations and constraints of the internal and external environments in which they operate. Sport management professors can lead discussions on the differences and similarities of the controllable and predictable internal environment while also contrasting the unpredictable external environment. Professors can focus on the tool of forecasting the changes they may confront. At this stage sport management students conduct a thorough SWOT analysis that details and describes the Strengths, Weaknesses, Opportunities, and Threats for the company and products.

Stage IV: Comprehensive review of the business plan. At this stage students ask for feedback regarding their work on the venture. Sport management professors can form in-class or online groups where at least two students review and comment on the work of the other students in the group. Then, students, based on the work from that exercise, write a review of which items need to be enhanced, changed, removed, or added to produce a quality and effective business plan.

As an alternative, students can select the type of research they would like to conduct in relation to the topic of business plan development. Students can select an existing company, create a new venture for an organization they are familiar with (internship, past or current employment site), or critique from the standpoint of a consultant and provide resources and information on how to enhance the existing documents.

Advanced Topics in Sport Management

One of the underlying questions that seems to surface in most sport management specific courses is what makes a sport organization successful? When we examine the sport management industry we can take a look further into the structure of sport. Students of sport management have a unique opportunity to analyze stand-alone sport companies, sport organizations that are affiliated with a league or conference, sport leagues that dominate our culture, and sport governing bodies at the national and international levels.

Activity I: Examining Leagues

Students compare and contrast, from an industry analyst perspective, for a number of leagues, including but not limited to the National Football League, National Hockey League, Major League Soccer, NASCAR, National Basketball Association, Professional Golfers' Association, and Ladies Professional Golf Association. Areas of concentration and study can be tailored by the sport management professor. **Table 4.1** lists the concepts students can investigate and explore.

Table 4.1 Sport Industry Analysis

- The make-up and structure of each league
- The similarities and differences between the leagues
- The strengths and weaknesses of the leagues (or complete SWOT analysis)
- The top identifiable valuable players of the league (sport)
- The issues or current trends (positive and negative) with the athletes of the league (sport)
- The type(s) of media attention focused on the league or sport or teams
- The target market, demographics, and psychographics of the core market for the league or sport
- The fan cost index for attendance at the sporting event
- Future direction of the league relating to rule changes, media contracts, player salary agreements, fan cost index, ownership structure, and sponsorships

---

Activity II: League Think

The sport management professor can discuss and ask students to probe specific details of each of the leagues and sport including:
- Revenue sharing
- Player contracts
- Revenues and expenditures
- Television contracts
- Features of stadium venue (plans for future expansion, parking, concessions, ticket availability)
- Changes in each of the leagues over last 2 years, 5 years, 10 years, 15 years, 20 years, and 30 years

Activity III: Comparison of National Versus International Leagues

Students can select one league in their home country and one international sport league to study. Students gain insight regarding the challenges of operating sport organizations domestically and abroad. Sport management professors can use this activity to encourage students to think about the economic opportunities and constraints, political issues in countries that may impede the enhancement of sport organizations, the role of governments in sport operations, and the difference in media attention and media access in different countries.

Questions to Consider

- Based on student interest in sport management, what kinds of practical assignments can you use in courses to investigate common challenges and opportunities in the financial landscape that is sport business management?
- What other tools can be explored in your courses to effectively prepare undergraduate and graduate sport management students entering a sport marketplace filled with economic uncertainty?
- What teaching methods will you adopt to assist students in gaining the requisite knowledge to understand the fundamental and core concepts associated with financial management?

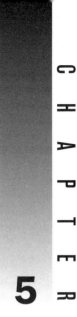

Teaching Activities: Sport Marketing and Sport Sponsorship

The sport management enterprise has created numerous opportunities for students to complete internships and become employed in the sport marketing setting of the industry. Often, sport management students begin their journey in sport management through entry-level positions in sport marketing departments for colleges, universities, or minor league and professional league sports. Sport marketing activities for sport organizations typically require enthusiastic and creative personnel who can connect with target groups. Students, to be effectively educated in sport marketing, need to be able to apply fundamental marketing principles to the unique aspects of the sport industry. Through the delivery of sport marketing courses and topics, educators can assist students in developing the requisite tools to handle the rigor and challenges associated with marketing sport in a competitive entertainment environment.

This chapter explores the following course objectives that can be embedded in assessment activities:
- Recognition and identification of sport as a product or service
- Dynamic relationship between sport and consumer buying behavior
- Analysis of sport and athletes as powerful selling tools
- Utilization of marketing and promotional techniques to develop sponsorship and fund-raising proposals and events

Sport Marketing Sectors of Sport Management

Discussion areas for the study of sport marketing revolve around marketing definitions, strategies, and research. It is important that sport management students understand the vital role of marketing within the sport industry. Marketing make take several forms for sport businesses. Students must be able to differentiate between the use of marketing to sell sport products and/or services from the use of sport and sport personality marketing to sell general or sport-related products and/or services.

Add to the sport marketing setting the role of professional athletes as product endorsers. Sport management students must grasp the wide-reaching capabilities of athletes who compete internationally versus domestically,

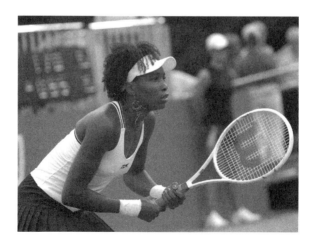

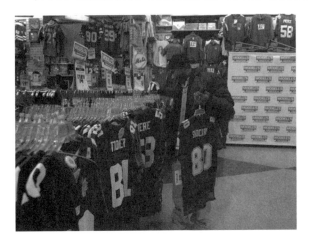

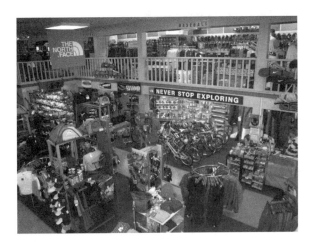

the perception of male and female professional athletes in their potential role as a product spokesperson, and the degree to which the type of sport plays in the visibility and appeal of professional athletes both internationally and domestically.

A central concept of sport marketing is sport sponsorship. Students, in this area of study, should be able to understand the rationale for corporations/businesses to spend resources to be somehow associated with a sporting event. On the other hand, students must also comprehend the importance of attracting and securing corporate sponsors for local, national, and international events.

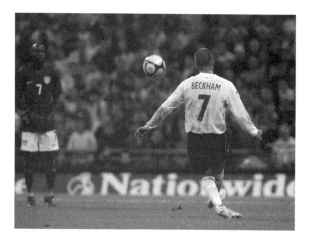

Activity I: Sport Product or Service Invention

To connect the discussion points of marketing to sport, students complete a comprehensive project that captures all elements of the marketing mix and marketing plan development. Early in the semester sport management educators can devote class discussions to the definition of sport marketing and the four or five elements of the marketing mix (product, price, place, promotion, and, if desired, public relations). For sport management professors to assess the knowledge accumulation of students in the area of sport marketing, the following project can be assigned.

Task 1: Students are asked to think about a sport product or service that could enhance or change an aspect of interest within the sport management industry. In the stage of brainstorming ideas for a new sport product or service, students are encouraged to reach out to others outside of the classroom for advice and feedback. Students develop a list of three potential ideas for approval by the instructor. The requirement is for students to create or invent a product or service that does not currently exist in the marketplace. Typically, some students generate ideas that are already established products on the market. Students are asked to thoroughly research their idea before submitting their list for approval. Over the years students have produced ideas that have the capability, viability, and sustainability of penetrating the marketplace. The students may need some direction and guidance early in the idea phase so they do not fall behind on the proceeding assignments and tasks.

Task 2: Once the final idea is approved, students write a clear and concise description of the product to share with their class mates. For traditional face-to-face class settings students can ask for feedback regarding their idea. In the online setting sport management professors can set up a discussion board or forum to generate the same type of response and feedback from students. Included in the description is the created name of the company that will ultimately produce the invention. The second part of this task is to name the product or service and with a stated product or service slogan. Finally, students identify one specific target market for their product.

Teaching Tip

Sport management professors can now address the issue of the importance of identifying a core market for a product or service. Often, students are not going to select a small and specific market for their product. Instead, students believe their product can be marketed and sold to broad and homogeneous groups of people with similar interests. For example, for students to grasp the idea of target market development, students can be assigned the task of researching one specific target market for one product currently in the market (**Figure 5.1**).

Teaching Tip

Does everyone really watch the Super Bowl? One leading question used in a sport marketing course is to provoke students to think beyond their personal feelings regarding sport or a sporting event. Many students believe the Super Bowl is a catch-all event and that "all" people are tuning in to watch the game. Is this fact or popular myth? Students can be assigned the duty of determining the market or markets of viewers and attendees for this major sporting event. After the research is collected, the sport management educator can spend time reviewing the definition and scope of target market development. In addition, students may come to the conclusion that perhaps events may attract a diverse group of markets

Figure 5.1 Target Market Development

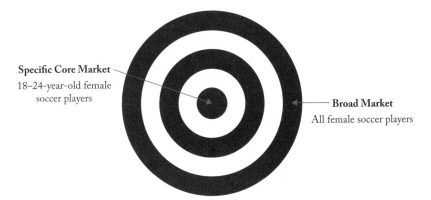

Specific Core Market
18–24-year-old female
soccer players

Broad Market
All female soccer players

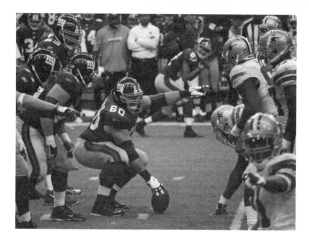

all with diverse needs and interests. For example, those who attend the game may attend for a variety of reasons. Some may be fans of the participating teams, whereas others may just be fans of football. Some sit in premium seats with higher costs than those seats located further away from the center of the field. There can also be a discussion regarding the viewers for this event. Some may watch just for the commercials, whereas some may watch because they enjoy each play of the game. What is important to note is that the sporting event attracts a number of people and fills a particular need or desire for those groups.

Task 3: Once students settle on one target market for their product idea the research stage begins. Students describe the target market using demographics (age, gender, income, education, sport preference). Sport management educators can assist students in breaking down the market demographics even further. For example, if a student plans to market a product for the sport of field hockey, the sport management professor can prompt the student to critically analyze details of their target market. The demographic breakdown for a field hockey market may include age, gender, level of play in the sport (recreation, high school, college; this can be broken down further into Division I, II, or III), years involved with sport (can be a numeric value or predetermined categories; novice, beginner, advanced), amount of money spent annually on the sport of field hockey (this may include fees, equipment, travel), number of days per week playing field hockey, and geographic location (East Coast, West Coast, or a specific region of the country, i.e., New York). Students then get a better sense of the scope and importance of developing and understanding target markets. The above listing of target market information includes not only demographic information but psychographic and geographic data regarding a target market.

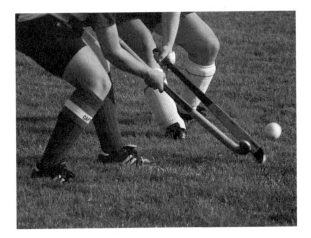

For this task students uncover as much information as possible from reliable sources to determine if this pool of individuals is a viable market for their product. From the collected research students can identify significant characteristics regarding their target market to aid in the process of creating and marketing the product. Students must convince the reader (instructor) that there is a need for their product from the perspective of the target market and that the need will be met by the product. Students create a written proposal (three pages) persuading the reader that the product features match the needs, wants, and desires of the stated target market. Using the collected research, students present their findings to the reader. Students may consider more than one market to research, which is fine; however, it is important that each student remains focused on one core group to satisfy the delivery of this product or service.

Task 4: What comes first, the product or the market? This is an interesting debate that can channel the students into thinking more about their idea and the marketplace they wish to enter. Of course, we need to think about consumers' needs for a particular product, and at the same time we may have a product that fills a newly created need for market. For this stage of the assignment students can start to focus on the special aspects of their product or service and how the product will succeed in the marketplace. Sport management professors can devote time discussing the reasons why new endeavors fail and others succeed by grasping the needs of consumer groups. Students are required to indicate how and why their product stands out against products that may already exist, any substitute products on the market (students need to understand that currently the target market(s) are using other products or services to fulfill a need), and how they will enter a congested marketplace with a new product.

Task 5: Meet with your class consultant. Each student can be randomly paired with any other student in the course to assist with getting feedback and guidance on the project. Students are asked to present their collection of information to their consultant either during or outside of class time. This same exchange can occur online using file sharing between consultants. Consultants are required to create a brief written report on the project they are critiquing; in return each student gets information to help fine-tune his or her product or service. This exercise helps both parties in gathering information and generating fresh ideas for their project. This collaborative activity allows students to "test" the marketplace to determine if they are heading in the right direction or if more time and resources are required to enhance the idea.

Teaching Tip

For team building in sport marketing, have each student select one or two other students in the class to be his or her consultant for in-class projects. Students while developing a new product or service have the chance to "bounce" ideas off their consultant as the project is being formulated. Professors can designate in-class time for students to spend communicating and learning from the feedback of their classroom consultant.

Task 6: Primary data from target markets is collected. At this stage students conduct a focus group to once again gather feedback and suggestions to adapt the product to fit into the marketplace. Students are asked to meet with a group of 4 to 10 members of their focus group at the same time in one meeting place. Often, students want to conduct one-on-one interviews, but this does not have the same effect of brainstorming and building on the comments of others as a focus group in one meeting place. If students are unable to gather members of their target market for reasons such as they are professional athletes or young children, sport management educators can direct students to meet with a group of people who may be able to respond like their target market would in similar situations. Before the focus group meeting students are required to submit a list of preset questions they wish to ask with the understanding they may need to ask follow-up or different questions that may not be on their original list due to the flow and progress of the meeting. Students take notes during the focus group meeting and submit a written review of the meeting. Within the written report students should include the true demographic information of the focus group and final conclusions and changes that may be made due to the ideas and feedback generated from the meeting.

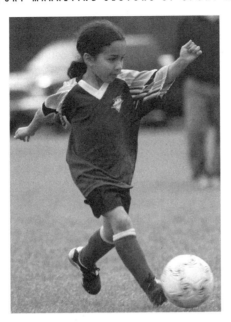

Task 7: At this point in the project development, students have a clear description of the product or service along with a specific target market. To effectively market the idea, students need to research the competition. How will a new product compete against existing and recognizable companies within the sport industry? Students research current companies that produce similar product lines or exist within a particular sport segment under which the newly created product falls. This portion of the project can include as much information as possible regarding competitor or substitute product target market(s), product cost, and channels of distribution for the product. From this information students can determine how they will effectively market their product, the potential selling price of the product, and methods for selling the product (retail store or online distribution channels as examples).

Task 8: Students probably have the most fun and creativity in completing a marketing and promotional campaign for the product. Students are asked to create a slogan for the product as early as Task 2 of the project. For this section students determine an effective message they would like to communicate to their designated target market. Students can rely once again on a focus group for feedback on the design of the campaign along with using the expertise of other faculty members on campus. The promotional campaign can take several forms, and students are encouraged to use a format and medium that most effectively accomplishes their goals.

Teaching Tip

Sport management professors can review the definition and components of a promotional campaign to launch a new product into the marketplace. Students need to consider all obstacles and opportunities that can exist when marketing a new product. At this point in the project students begin to realize all previously completed work will assist them in properly and effectively meeting the needs of their identified consumer group.

Task 9: After students have collected information and made adjustments to their original idea, students present the product to the class. Students have 4 minutes to convince and persuade the audience (who will be acting as the identified target market) if the product or service will have a chance to succeed in the sport marketplace.

Task 10: At the conclusion of the project students reflect on the series of tasks completed over several weeks of the semester. Students are directed to comment on what worked and what did not work in the process of developing a new product for a new target group. In addition, students provide insight as to what components of the marketing plan they needed to spend more time developing. Each student collects feedback through the online forum from each of his or her course mates regarding the potential success of the idea and comments for improvements.

Teaching Tip

As a method to explain strategic planning from a marketing perspective, sport management educators can explore a mock company to communicate the requisite components. Sport management educators can select any type of product or service to assist in the comprehension and application of sport marketing tools. The new company is Gentile In-Line Skates with the primary product to be marketed "in-line skates or roller blades." Students are prompted to discuss the growth potential (if any) of this product and the potential marketplace. Using a simple graphic pie chart (**Figure 5.2**), students are directed to consider all of types of consumer groups who may purchase Gentile In-Line Skates.

Figure 5.2 Breaking Down Target Groups

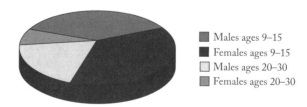

- Males ages 9–15
- Females ages 9–15
- Males ages 20–30
- Females ages 20–30

From the large circular graph students may argue that children (both boys and girls) and adults (both men and women) may be potential Gentile In-Line Skate consumers. The sport management professor can then extract more information regarding the target market by asking a series of questions (**Table 5.1**) regarding the demographics of the target market.

The more layers of questions that can be injected into the discussion, the closer the class/group will get to the identification of the core target market. The sport management professor can then connect the opening discussion to the larger point of strategic planning in sport management. Students, using Gentile In-Line Skates, can apply the role of strategic planning and the elements of strategic planning for practical purposes. The following elements can be found under this discussion activity:

- *Mission statement development:* Most students have gained knowledge and experience reviewing and developing mission statements in previous classes. Students can be directed to research mission statements from other sport-related businesses to understand the scope and purpose of the statement.

Table 5.1 Breaking Down Target Groups

- Who would consume this sport-related product?
- Who would be interested and/or desire using this sport-related product?
- How can we make the potential market aware of this sport-related product?
- Who has the purchasing power to participate in the exchange process?
- What are the demographics and psychographics of the core market?
- How many times per week, per season, and per year would the core market use this sport-related product?
- How much money may they spend on this sport-related product?
- How can we create interest in a cluttered marketplace for this new sport-related product?
- What tangible benefits will the core market seek by using this sport-related product?
- Where would this group most likely purchase this (online or retail stores)?
- How can your company meet the needs of the market while fulfilling your goals and objectives?

- *Organizational objectives:* The class can identify measurable outcomes for the new company and the new product over the business cycle. An example may be to capture 5% of the target market. Objectives can be considered the pathways or map to assist in the achievement of goals that are specific to the sport company.
- *Organizational strategies:* For Gentile In-Line Skates to be successful in the marketplace, strategies need to be discussed and clarified. Sport management professors can review the definitions of each of these components along with providing concrete examples of the target market and product for the following available strategies: market penetration, market development, product development, and diversification.

Activity II: Sport Sponsorship Event Creation From Start to Finish

For students to get a sense of what it takes to create and organize an event, professors can incorporate an activity called "From Start to Finish." The sport management instructor selects events that currently exist: Division I Softball World Series, NCAA Fencing Championship, Preseason Kickoff Celebration, or Midnight Madness: Basketball Blastoff. Students form groups to appropriately tackle the components of their designated event. Students need to create this event (on paper) from start to finish. Students are to act in the role of sponsorship director and event coordinator.

The "From Start to Finish" components are as follows:

1. Students select a future date and location for the event.
2. Students consider all tasks that need to be accomplished to make the event a success.
3. Students consider all responsibilities and duties of the various sport managers of the organizations.
4. Students start to research the actual event to determine their needs for a future event.
5. Students are asked to think about job titles and create job descriptions for each of their group members. Professors can work with students in the development of specific and accurate responsibilities for their designated event.
6. From the job descriptions students create an organizational chart and reporting structure.
7. Students then create a marketing piece for the event. The purpose of the media publication is to promote and create an awareness of the event.
8. Students present their "From Start to Finish" project to the class for feedback and evaluation.

This project simulates the stages of developing an actual sport management event. Sport management educators assign students to research profit or nonprofit events throughout the duration of the activity. Topics that can be further explored through readings and supplemental lectures include chain of command, hierarchical structure, job description creation, the hiring process, phases of organizational control, delegating, and accountability.

Activity III: Sport Promotion Success or Failure

Students are guided to select an article relating to a promotional event that was either a success or failure. The written portion of the assignment includes information regarding the company/event during the time of the promotional campaign being addressed, other promotional campaigns (past and or present created for the company), facts regarding the promotion, rationale for adopting the promotion, and result of promotion (success or failure). Each student gets the opportunity to present his or her promotion to the class for review and analysis. Students should be prepared to respond to any questions and to pose one to two follow-up questions from the perspective of sport marketing consultants.

Teaching Tip

Sport management professors can lead a lecture discussion on the role of promotions in sport management, promotions defined, types of promotional campaigns, and the process of developing and creating promotional campaigns.

Teaching Tip

For online or hybrid courses students can link the article for the sport promotion that is reviewed for the assignment. Students can post their written analysis along with responses to follow-up questions asked by course mates. In addition, students may also post related links to add depth to the online discussion board or forum.

Activity IV: Sport Personalities and Marketing

Students research a sport personality (coach, athlete, sport broadcaster, sport marketer) who has made a significant impact on sport business. Students report on the contribution and ideals this person injected into their particular sport and beyond. Students indicate what they have learned from their discovery of information and how they will apply that knowledge and information in sport marketing.

Activity V: Impact of Sport Products on the Industry

Students research and select a sport product or service that has changed the sport industry in either a positive or negative light. For example, for the 2006–2007 National Basketball Association season a new and improved ball was introduced in the league. The effects of the new ball were not positive, and many argued it changed the nature of the game and the performances of the athletes. After a few weeks the ball was replaced by the original ball due to many complaints by National Basketball Association players. Students can present their findings orally or electronically to course mates. To get a large pool of ideas, students should not duplicate the selection of others.

Teaching Tip

Sport management faculty can discuss the type of individual or product appropriate for the activity. Students often select a sport icon that is commonly discussed. Perhaps students can go back in time to pick a sport product or person from a particular decade.

Activity VI: Change the School Mascot

Many college and universities have used sport team mascots to get fans excited about games. Sport mascots at the professional and collegiate levels have in recent times received media attention for their on-field and off-field antics. Students are charged with either changing their school mascot or enhancing the school mascot. Sport management professors can also direct students to create an entire college-wide celebration to introduce the new and/or improved mascot to the college community while also promoting their sport teams. A series of discussions can be conducted outside of the classroom to determine the necessary means to enhance the visibility of the mascot and connect the mascot excitement to increased awareness of sport teams on campus. Students should be able to articulate their plan to increase attendance based on the launching of a new athletic mascot.

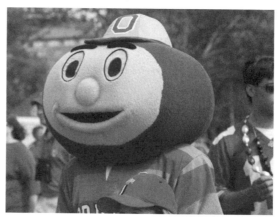

Activity VII: Adopt a Team

Students in a sport marketing course are challenged to increase attendance at games for one assigned sport team on campus. Students are asked to create a promotional campaign to attract a new fan base to a team in need. Often, on a college campus some teams naturally have a larger fan base than other teams. Students have the opportunity to discuss the reasons why students do or do not attend certain sporting events. In the process students become more familiar with each team with which they are affiliated, and from that they can develop a marketing plan with the one goal to increase on-campus attendance at events. This is a practical activity, and students can immediately determine the results of their efforts. Discussions can focus on times of the events, competing campus-wide events, cost of attendance of events, accessibility of parking near the athletic venue, and satisfaction of supporting the college team.

Activity VIII: Advertisements and Sport: An Interactive Project

Sport management professors conduct an online sport marketing and sponsorship activity. Students are responsible for discussing and interacting with course mates through the course website or designated online medium. Professors organize a course online during a televised sporting event such as the Super Bowl, Olympics, World Cup, or NASCAR events. Professors can set up their online course information detailing the requirements of the work during the televised or web-casted event. Using the course websites, professors can hold live chats and at the same time use discussion boards to facilitate the discussions on hand. Topics can range from sponsorship, to commercials, to event management, to fan analysis, to sport spectatorship, to ambush marketing. Students can interactively participate as the event is being broadcast. This type of activity places the students at the center of the event and creates a distinguishing perspective that cannot be simulated in the traditional classroom setting.

Students are required to watch the event live and participate in the work through the course website simultaneously as the event is being aired. Students discuss, in live time, the designated discussion points and others that may be generated through the circumstances created during the event.

Teaching Tip

As students watch the televised/web-streamed event they keep a log of sponsors associated with the event, companies, products, and target markets for the advertisements. The target market(s) for the event can be identified and analyzed as well. This discussion could occur before the event, and then this exercise can be an affirmation of their findings.

1. What is the purpose of advertising during the Super Bowl (or designated sporting event)?
2. Does the final score (or win–loss records of the participating teams) play a role in the viewership of the commercials or the effectiveness of sponsorship opportunities?
3. Which companies should have saved their financial resources and avoided marketing at the designated event?
4. For the Super Bowl activity, the following are some questions that can be implemented into the activity:
   - Why do Super Bowl commercials get so much attention?
   - Is there another sporting event that can come close to the Super Bowl and the cost for airing commercials?
   - What is the incentive for television networks to promote upcoming shows during sporting events? Does that have a positive effect on future viewership?

After the half of the Super Bowl (or designated point of the televised event), students can be assigned to groups (by company associated with the event) to continue studying the companies, target markets, and products associated with the sporting event. Students are required to determine and present

1. Company mission statement
2. Advertising theme and target market
3. Product line (all) of the companies associated with the event
4. Why is the company invested in advertising time during the game?
5. Whether the money spent for the advertisement(s) was well spent (include research and data to support response)
6. Whether any changes occurred since the event (via company website)
7. Whether the company received new visitors to their site due to the event
8. Their ranking of commercials (top three favorite commercials from a fan's perspective, top three favorite commercials from a sport management executive perspective, least effective commercial from a fan's perspective, and least effective commercial from a sport management executive perspective)
9. Trends that may or may not exist in the types of companies that are associated with the event
10. Themes that exist in the commercials associated with the event (Do these themes remain the same from year to year or change?)

Activity IX: Charitable Causes and Sport

A variety of relationships exists between sport team and charities. Students study the purpose of developing these exchange relationships between sport and charities. A dialogue can center on the benefits sport organizations receive from their involvement and contributions (financial) to charitable causes. Sport management students can select one team or league to determine the scope of their activities with giving. Some examples of charitable connections with sport teams include United Way and the Jimmy Fund.

Activity X: Creation of a New Intramural League

Intramurals and recreational leagues are both popular and common across college and university campuses. Students enjoy the refreshing and non-competitive environment offered by recreational programs. Often, students have ideas for implementing or including new sports and leagues to recreational offerings. Through this activity students develop and create a new intramural league on campus. Students create promotional literature regarding the league, write a sport story about the new league for inclusion in the school newspaper, and create the sport league schedule, rules, fees, and awards. Students present their creation to a mock student development committee for feedback. Students play dual roles in the activity as creators of the new league and then again as members of the student development committee.

Activity XI: Online Discussion Board Technology

The methods for promoting and marketing sport services and products are evolving at a rapid pace. In this activity students begin to discover the technological and electronic advancements in sport management and sport marketing. Students select an article that discusses emergent technology, such as viral marketing and social networking connections that sport management professionals can use to attract consumers and secure advertisers. Students are asked to post the information and the article link within the course discussion board. To spark a discussion students can pose two or three follow-up questions for course mates to respond, debate, and argue.

Activity XII: Student Summary and Thoughts

To assess and collect information regarding student learning, sport management professors can distribute an informal evaluation of the course while also responding to pertinent course concepts. This activity can be attached to a graded assignment or just used as a final assessment piece for the course. This listing of questions can also be adapted to be used for a variety of sport management courses:

1. What did you learn or gain from your participation in the course?
2. Did you enjoy the online format? Please explain.
3. What topics will you continue to explore due to the course activities?
4. Please respond in your own words and using the knowledge gained from the course to the following (five-paragraph minimum):
   • What is sport marketing?
   • What is the importance of market research?
   • What is the relationship between sport, promotions, marketing, sponsorships, and consumers?
5. What are the key features of sport marketing that will sustain sports into the future based on the work of the class (two paragraphs)?
6. If you were teaching the course, how would you explain the elements of the marketing mix for a sport-specific company? You select the company/product and educate the teacher on the marketing mix.
7. In developing a marketing plan, why is the SWOT (Strengths, Weaknesses, Opportunities, and Threats) analysis an essential part of the process? Please relate your response to the current marketplace.
8. What grade do you believe you earned in the course? Why?

Activity XIII: Careers in Sport Marketing

The vast number of career opportunities that exist in the sport marketing sector can be presented to students through the discovery process. Students, through this exercise, are expected to list and describe the roles and career opportunities that exist in sport marketing. Students then articulate either orally or electronically their selections to share with the class. Each of the roles and titles should also include a comprehensive description of the responsibilities of the position. Some lists that may be generated by students include the following positions in the sport marketing arena:

- Sport information director
- Sport marketing executives
- Sport promotions
- Sport sponsorship
- Hospitality management
- Event management
- Publicity services

- Public relations
- Cause sponsorship
- Community relations
- Sport agency

Activity XIV: Branding and Slogan Competition

Through this exercise students gain an appreciation of the importance of branding in the sport marketplace. The ultimate goal of any company is to instill an image, logo, or slogan into the minds of consumer groups. Consumers connect the brand to the quality of products or product lines. An engaging activity allows students to work in groups to come up with a list of sport-related company products or services and slogans that can identify the brand. The students have 5 minutes to generate a comprehensive list indicating product and slogan. One student represents each group in presenting the list to the class. The format is a "read off" whereby students line up in the front of the class. The first student lists on company and one slogan and then we move to the next student. The last student presents two companies and two slogans and we move back from the end of the line to the start. The last standing student and his or her group win. The other group members act as judges as the activity is being played. Students cannot wrongly communicate the product and/or slogan (if they do they are removed from the competition), and students cannot repeat a company or slogan that has already been used.

Activity XV: Create a Publicity Campaign

In some sport marketing courses students can work on developing writing and communicating skills through creating a publicity campaign for an athlete or team. Professors can have a preset list of potential athletes or teams for which students research and develop a campaign. In addition, professors can indicate the direction or impact the campaign should address. Students develop a theme or themes for the campaign, timeline for the delivery of media spots or opportunities for which the person or team would be required to perform, marketing pieces to inform companies and possible outlets regarding the athlete or team, and a written press release to communicate the efforts of the campaign. A second layer to this activity involves students in creating an actual press conference for the athlete or team. Students are responsible for selecting the appropriate venue and communicating (through a press release) the purpose of the press conference.

Activity XVI: Professional Athletes and Endorsements

In this exercise students are asked to create the perfect athlete in the realm of product endorsements. Sport management professors can lead a discussion on the various characteristics and attributes that assist athletes in secure endorsement deals. The components to be investigated while studying the relationship between athletes and endorsements are

- Image
- Appeal
- Product connection
- International versus domestic reach and appeal

Students can be directed to think in broad terms when considering athletes to be connected to sport products. To understand the fundamental elements of selecting professional athletes from a corporate perspective, students can research both company and athlete of an existing endorsement relationship to uncover the common characteristics of both the brand and the athlete.

Questions to Consider

- What activities could you incorporate into sport management courses to teach students to appreciate and understand the value and importance of market research?
- How can students be instructed to critically analyze the pricing decisions associated with marketing and ultimately selling sport products and/or services?
- Various and unique distribution methods exist for making sport related products available to the general public. What elements of product distribution will you incorporate into your lectures and discussions to allow students to determine and assess the best channels of distribution for sport-specific products or services?

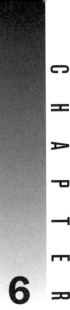

C
H
A
P
T
E
R

6

International Perspective on Sport Management

Sport as an entity sits in the global marketplace. Events like the Olympics and World Cup of Soccer and other sports draw fans and spectators from all continents. These global events have the capability of connecting people from different regions of the world to focus on sport. Sport is unique in that the power derived from its reach is unmatched by any other entertainment or business industry. Sport management students must comprehend and recognize the role of sport business in the global marketplace. To effectively prepare students to enter the international sport landscape, it is essential that sport management programs devote course time and material to teaching and assessing student learning in this dynamic growth area in sport management.

Content areas explored in this chapter include:
• Sport in the global landscape
• Sport products in the international marketplace
• Study of professional sport from an international perspective

Case Study Analysis

Perhaps the most effective teaching methodology that can be used to address the issues of sport from an international perspective is through current case study materials. Sport management professors can continue to provide information and insight through lectures and shared information. Case study utilization places our students in the role as decision maker for a particular company, event, or cause as it relates to sport in the global/international marketplace. Through case study preparation students are able to understand the tools and competencies required to make decisions that impact sport organizations. Sport management students apply theory to practice through the case scenario incorporated into course activities. Sport management students can contribute meaningful ideas and creative solutions to "real" scenarios and situations in sport business.

Professors can create their own case study based on experience with a particular organization or event. Effective case studies should provide the reader with background information regarding the organization, the current situation confronting the sport executive, and possible questions/concepts to the reader should explore and answer when creating a response

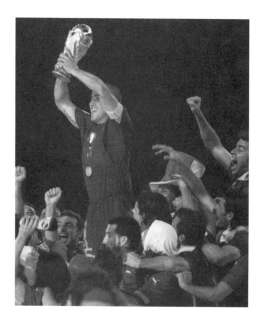

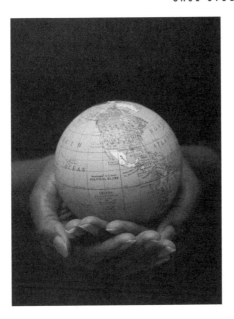

to the case study material. Sport management professors can use the *Harvard Business Review*, which offers volumes of sport management–specific case studies that can be purchased online by students. The selection of case studies ranges in topic, and the professor can select which case studies best fit the course.

Activity I: Journal Presentation—Global Landscape Q & A

Using a reference sport management journal, students select an article of their choice to educate the class on the topical issue. Students must relate the article to topical discussion points covered in the course. To effectively share information with other students, each student reviews the article and provides a visual presentation that can be posted online or presented as an in-class assignment. In both scenarios student presenters share the collected information, include teaching points regarding the subject matter to the class, and offer the class three questions for further inquiry and discussion. Students in this forum act as both learner and educator when responding to the statements and postings of others.

Activity II: International Marketplace

Students in this activity use their management skills and knowledge to create an international business opportunity for a domestic company aiming to enter the global marketplace.

Stage I: Students research domestic companies in the sport management industry. From the list of companies students can determine if one of the company products can be suitable, viable, and sustainable for international sales and marketing.

Stage II: Students must select the country in which the existing product will be marketed and eventually sold. Students compose an international marketplace report that addresses the following areas:

- *Introduction:* Historical/background information on the specific country
- *Scanning the environment:* Descriptions of cultural trends, customs, and unique traditions of the country that may impact marketing, advertising, and sales
- *Economic system:* Review of the financial markets, currency, and trade policies

Stage III: Once a country is selected students can begin to research the target groups for the particular product to be sold abroad. In addition, students identify the specific characteristics of the marketplace and the trends that may support sales of the product in the designated country.

Stage IV: Students examine marketing concepts used domestically and determine how, and if, those campaigns need to be adapted to fit the international marketplace.

Stage V: At the conclusion of the project students present their information to the class. The form of the presentation should be a combination of a written proposal, audio-visual presentation (in class or online), and a Q & A forum to ascertain if in fact the idea is sustainable based on the comments of course mates for the international marketplace.

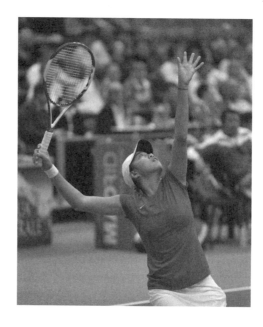

Stage VI: Synthesis and analysis. To learn from the feedback of others, students write a report analyzing the feedback and ideas gathered through the presentation. Students reflect on what changes they would make to their proposal based on the comments of others.

Activity III: Globalization of Professional Sport

Sport management courses may include some discussion regarding elements of sport in the global marketplace. To provide breadth to this area, the following topics can be explored in a stand-alone course or embedded into course content. Professional sport organizations are continually seeking diverse opportunities to reach a larger base of consumers (which can prove to be a lucrative decision). Students can be assigned to study and research the marketing efforts and global initiatives associated with the following professional sport organizations:

- National Basketball Association
- National Football League
- Major League Soccer
- Major League Baseball
- Professional Golfers' Association
- Ladies Professional Golf Association

Stage I: Research Paper

Students are asked to write a paper from the perspective of a sport business consultant or executive. Students can report on the current activities as they relate to the global initiatives along with practical suggestions for outreach and marketing to different target groups in an international capacity. In addition, students can be assigned to compare their league research with one other league to determine, in terms of global and international reach, which league has the best chance to succeed in the new marketplace.

Stage II: Consulting Presentation

Based on the research students are asked to formally present their findings along with the current situational analysis of the sport entity they have studied. Students must provide facts regarding the current initiative of the company, goals for international expansion for the company, and tangible methods for achieving or enhancing their global reach and positioning in the international sport marketplace. Once the student has presented their information, the audience is free to ask follow-up questions. Students, acting as consultants, are encouraged to professionally address each question or concern presented by course mates. Students can be evaluated on their written, verbal, and critical analysis through this activity.

Activity IV: Debates

As companies seek to expand their reach and enter the global marketplace, many challenges and concerns become topics for debate in the college classroom. Some critical decisions large and recognizable sport companies make have come under scrutiny by the media and human rights activists. Some topics to be explored include

- Outsourcing
- Olympic sport
- Sport governance
- Human rights and sport management
- Internet broadcasting and the international marketplace

Teaching Tip

Sport management professors have the option to integrate web-based tools to create a dynamic teaching and learning environment using a debate forum by using a course blog. Some course management programs at institutions already have blog capabilities as a feature of the course management system. If professors would like to create their own blog space they may consider many free blog resources that exist online, such as pbwiki.com.

Blog Setup

Professors begin the process by selecting a debate topic to explore with the class (e.g., International Sourcing: Nike and Reebok). Students can participate as individuals or assigned groups for the blog exercise. Blogs can be a unique way for students to share their thoughts on a topic, receive feedback from others in the course, and continue the discourse at higher levels of thinking and analysis. Students can also be required to find, share, summarize, and cite two to three reference articles or resources to support their perspective and add evidence to their position on the issue.

Stage I: The sport management professor presents the debate topic and the question(s) to be explored over a designated time period.

Stage II: Each student or student group adds their opening perspective or statement on the issue to start the blog debate.

Stage III: Students must be made aware of the amount of time and quantity of blog entries that are acceptable for their participation in the blog over the designated time period.

Stage IV: Students should be prompted by course mates or the professor to critically analyze the debate questions through follow-up questions and further inquiry on the topic.

Stage V: Each student or student group at the close of the blog exercise enters their final viewpoint on the issue based on the learning and sharing of information that was part of the blog.

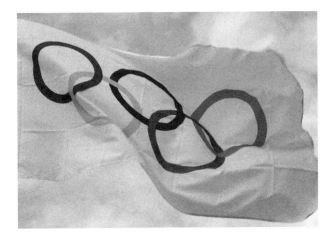

Questions to Consider

- What resources can you incorporate into your courses to investigate and explore the global impact of sport?
- Create a list of domestic companies that have an international marketing reach in sport management and sport business. What features of these companies could you discuss in class when covering sport in the global marketplace?
- Which country or countries are the best marketplaces for international alliances and expansion of sport leagues, sales of sport products, or sales of sport services?

Legal Aspects of Sport

Most sport management programs of study use a stand-alone course that tackles the elements and contents of legal issues in sport. Many sport management educators may dedicate class assignments and lectures on sport law–related topics within the courses they teach. Sport law and the legal issues associated with law are broad topics that require care when delivering the materials and information to students. Often, many sport management professors teaching these courses are not trained legal professionals; however, many have experienced the administrative and leadership side of managing issues that develop from a sport law perspective.

This chapter examines:

- The connection between theory and practical application of legal aspects of sport
- Teaching methodology used to capture the essence of sport law topics

Legal Aspects

Activity I: Competency Statements

Competency statements can be used in a number of courses and may also be included in the creation of student portfolios. In essence, competency statements (two to three paragraphs) are written explanations of sport law principles or concepts investigated throughout a given period of time. The construction of competency statements allows students to demonstrate their proficiency in the legal application of sport topics. After a reading in risk management, for example, students can connect and synthesize the information read with the generated discourse created from a previous lecture or class discussion. Students can then capture the competency (skill development and critical thinking) required for sport managers dealing with the issue of risk management in the sport business industry. Students can be assigned to write a number of competency statements throughout the semester. The culminating activity is to create a sport law professional portfolio developed from the collection of written competency statements captured throughout the semester.

Teaching Tip

Here is a student guide to developing competency statements.

1. Clearly introduce the topic. Include definitions and/or overview of specific legal case/scenario.
2. Describe from a sport management perspective how to apply the acquired concepts and information.
3. Provide a personal descriptive of the legal issue/concepts through work- or internship-related experiences.
4. Research and summarize a current article that directly relates to the topic and sport management.

Activity II: Sport Law Professional Portfolio

From the collection of sport law competency statements and other material(s) from the course, legal concepts and their application can be further explored and analyzed to develop a sport law professional portfolio. For the sport law professional portfolio, students, at the preliminary stage, introduce the objectives of the sport law course to the reader. Next, students describe how the sport law course has helped them to become a better sport management practitioner. Students, based on their area of interest in the discipline, communicate the methods used in the course to apply legal concepts to specific sport management situations. Using readings, projects, and assignments students describe their professional development in learning and applying legal principles to the sport management setting.

Sport and Law Today

Students are asked to create a list of issues under the heading of legal aspects of sport for this assignment. The list is class generated and shared with the group. Students then select one topic for further study that is presented to the class.

Activity III: Topics of Study in the Legal Domain

Students collect five research articles on the designated topic along with two to three newsworthy articles from the popular media. Each student is responsible for submitting a four-page paper to the professor along with presenting the material to the class using the course website or a traditional in-class presentation. Students present a lecture-formatted presentation with the sole purpose of educating classmates on the topic at hand. Students are required to engage the class in dialogue and discussion along with presenting material that is content focused. At the conclusion of the presentation students pose three questions for the class to respond to and/or to be included in a subsequent examination in the class.

Activity IV: Legal Debates

For selected and designated weeks in the course, the sport management professor can organize debate topics for students to explore in the field of sport law. Students present their position and perspective on a variety of topics along with posting additional resources within the course website. Students read the work of others, probe, and respond on the designated forum created on the course website. From the online starting point, the debate and discussion can then continue and be amplified within the traditional classroom setting.

Additionally, sport management professors can designate a role for each person in the course to create positions and perspectives for the debate. An interesting component is that students may be asked to be for or against a topic even though they may have the opposing viewpoint. In this environment students are forced to execute a debate perspective that is outside their comfort zone and belief system. This approach encourages open minds, critical thinking, and an appreciation of diverse viewpoints.

Activity V: Legal Case Study Debates

For this activity students in one class are assigned a legal case study to create discussion, analysis, and debate on the issue(s). Students are assigned to the following groups:
- Plaintiffs
- Defendants
- Judges (they decide based on the presented positions which direction to rule)

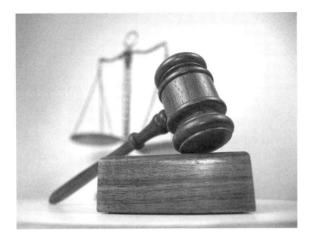

From the designated case study, students present opening arguments regarding the legal issue at hand. Students are required to find other cases that are similar in nature in which students can use to support their arguments.

The following guide is used when analyzing the case law:

1. *Facts:* Each student determines what is relevant in terms of the legal aspects of the case.
2. *Issues:* Students must clearly define the issue of the case (e.g., negligence, wrongful termination, breach of contract).
3. *Rulings:* Students research other cases and determine how the court ruled (in favor of plaintiff or defendant).
4. *Rationale:* Based on the ruling, students indicate the reason and rationale for the decision of the court.

Activity VI: Legal Brief

Students are required to compose a legal brief consistent with the arguments presented within the case. Students must include the essential facts of the case, statement of the question of law involved in the case, methods of applying the law, and the arguments used in similar cases and circumstances. In addition, students devise, from a sport management or administrative perspective, a comprehensive plan to prevent the legal issue from surfacing once again in the workplace.

Activity VII: Research in Sport Law

For students to gain a greater appreciation of the vast topics of study in sport law, sport management professors can require students to research topics and share the research with classmates. Some critical and timely topics in sport law are listed in **Table 7.1**.

Table 7.1 Research Topics in Sport Law

- Governing structure of sports (regulations, sanctions, membership, control)
- National Collegiate Athletic Association compliance issues and concerns (athlete eligibility, drug testing)
- Liability of coaches, officials, and independent contractors
- Risk management and crisis planning
- Role of the athletic trainer in the competitive sport setting
- Discrimination issues (Title IX)
- Collective bargaining in sport
- Fantasy sport and new domain of legal concerns
- Sport agency

The list provided in Table 7.1 shows examples of research topics. The list can evolve and change as the interests of the students differ from semester to semester. Sport management professors can develop examination questions from the student-driven presentations that can tap into the student's knowledge base and comprehension of legal concepts.

Activity VIII: Sport Governing Bodies

Sport governance impacts the organization and management of sport across the globe. Sport management students should gain an understanding of local, national, and international associations that create policy, guidelines, and regulations for sport programs and offerings. Students select one governing body to study for the assignment.

Stage I: The governing body is selected.

Stage II: The research for this assignment is centered in educating course mates on the mission, role, and governing reach of the specific sport association. Students are required to research the history and current situation of the sport governance association.

Stage III: Students are to report any minor or major rules, regulations, or changes that have occurred over the last decade in the association.

Stage IV: The final report and presentation allows students to communicate the process of discovery working with the information of the sport governance association along with some essential information to share with the class.

Activity IX: Sport Governance Research

Students, for this exercise, are to select a topic that is related to the governance of sport. To elimination duplication of the type of governing body being studied, the topic should be approved by the sport management professor in advance. Students should be directed to also research a topic within the study that must involve sport economics and legal practices as it relates to various sport governance issues. In addition, it should be data driven, meaning students conduct research in collecting quantitative and/or qualitative information on the topic.

Teaching Tip

Here are tips for creating a sport governance research paper:
- *Introduction*: Professors should spend time in class and perhaps during office hours to assist students in developing a specific question to be explored with the research. Students should answer the following: what are you trying to enhance or improve through the sport governance research initiative?
- *Argument*: Students should be poised to communicate what elements or features distinguish their paper from others.
- *Audience*: To present students with a focus target group when writing the paper, it makes sense to have students communicate what group of people would benefit the most from reading this paper.

Questions to Consider

- Title IX has been a major focus area for sport law courses. What teaching methods and activities can you incorporate into your course to assist students in tracing the historical aspects of this legislation and determining the effects of the legislation on athletics?
- Sport agency and the role of sport agents in sport is a recurring theme in sport law and administration courses. What activities and/or sources will you use to assist students in critically analyzing the impact (positive/negative) sport agency has played on intercollegiate athletics and professional sports?
- What projects and assignments can students complete to have an understanding and appreciation of various legal rulings and their connection to the sport industry?

Teaching With Technology

In recent years embracing and integrating technology into the sport management classroom has become a major thrust for colleges and universities. Many institutions are looking to gain competitive advantages in the recruitment of students by promoting and marketing state-of-the-art technology on campus. Many in sport management have experience using mediated (any multimedia equipment, from overhead projector to DVD player) classrooms. Many, if not all, in sport management have used "smart boards," which allow professors to present lectures in dynamic fashion and write on computer screens during lectures. Although these programs create a classroom filled with technology, the lingering question remains: Does technology enhance student learning?

This chapter examines:
- Academic technology in the sport management curriculum
- Integration of technology in the teaching classroom
- Implementation of the electronic portfolio within the sport management program of study

Technology and Sport Management

As institutions of higher education push forward on technology use and integration (over and beyond the basic use of slideshow lectures), many issues and concerns are presented to faculty members and administrators. The integration of technology into the academic classroom can be simply defined as using technology to improve or enhance the educational process. In our efforts to teach more effectively and enhance student learning, sport management educators need to make certain that the use of technology enhances classroom instruction and student learning. Virtual classrooms, where we never meet our students yet we deliver an academic experience that is both enriching and challenging, are today commonplace in higher education. Before moving forward on the complete integration of technology, sport management departments need to conduct a comprehensive and thorough review of the availability of academic technology, support systems for faculty and students, and the proper delivery of academic technology within the classroom setting and through online and hybrid courses.

Throughout the process of moving into a new way of teaching on campus, many find that faculty members may be uncomfortable with the use of technology as a teaching agent. Sport management administrators must consider a process whereby support can be provided for faculty members who need assistance integrating new media into their classroom delivery of course materials. Some institutions may designate a faculty mentor (mentors may already exist informally) who spends time troubleshooting or educating other faculty members throughout the semester. Sport management administrators must create a culture of sharing and helping so that the combination of technology and teaching does not turn into "survival of the technologically fit." Sport management administrators should be concerned that some faculty members will be left behind; for those not taking advantage of technology, are there consequences in their class evaluations impacting and affecting both merit and/or tenure?

With that being said, this is where the collaboration piece comes into place when dealing with integrating technology across the major or program of study. One solution is to connect with faculty members in other areas of studies and whose majors already have progressed forward on the technology initiative. Departments of sport management and its faculty members should be guided to cultivate relationships with those faculty members who have experience with incorporating new technology tools into their teaching toolbox.

Ultimately, sport management programs strive to demonstrate that the use of technology enhances student learning and effectively prepares students as they enter the professional/corporate setting. Integration of technology into the classroom forces not only students but faculty to step out of their comfort zones. For this reason we need to offer and provide a series of support programs to ease both groups into the process. **Table 8.1** reviews the questions to consider for the improvement of the learning environment when incorporating new media and technology into the classroom setting.

Sport management educators may want to determine what impact the use of this technology has on their students: Does the technology make the course better or worse? For all programs seeking accreditation from Commission on Sport Management Accreditation (COSMA), it is important to stay true to the created standards and to closely examine each course we teach to determine the appropriate times and topics to incorporate while using technology (**Table 8.2**).

Table 8.1 Academic Technology Integration

- Why teach with technology?
- What are the expectations of our students?
- What types of support structures exist at our institutions or within our sport management departments?
- What is the vision of the institution for academic technology across the curriculum and within sport management?

Table 8.2 Integration Checklist

- Where do we begin (or continue) to "integrate" technology into the sport management classroom?
- What are our comfort levels with technology?
- What do our supervisors/academic deans require for technology integration?
- How do we revise our syllabus to reflect the technology initiative?
- Where can you use or integrate technology based on an evaluation of courses?
- Where can technology improve student acquisition of knowledge?
- How can technology resources support student learning?
- How can we determine the value of the use of technology through assignments and course activities?

Educational technology can be described as "any means of communicating with learners other than through direct, face to face, or personal contact" (Bates & Poole, 2003, p. 5). This may include desktop computer to desktop computer utilization, web-enhanced coursework, instructional software, and video conferencing. Sport management academicians can use educational technology to build teaching tools and to captivate students in the learning process (**Table 8.3**). Educational technology can be useful in creating interactive learning activities within courses. These interactive experiences have the teaching power to enhance classroom discussion and to engage students, which improves the learning process (Gilbert & Moore, 1998).

Electronic Portfolio Implementation

Over the years in higher education, faculty and academic administrators searched and continue to search to find a tool that can assist in assessing and evaluating learning. One method of systematically requiring professors and students to create, store, and analyze educational materials is through portfolio development. The portfolio has often been used as a collection of designated pieces of work (**Box 8.1**). Portfolio use in higher education is not a new method of assessment, but the way we can deliver, compose, and evaluate the material has dramatically advanced.

BOX (**8.1**) **Definition: e-Portfolio.**

Systematic collections of student work selected to provide information about students' attitudes and motivation, level of development, and growth over time (Kingore, 1993).

Table 8.3 Integration Tips

- Identify the WHERE (which sport management courses?)
- Identify the WHEN (one assignment, semester long, project duration?)
- Identify the HOW (projects, assignments, e-portfolio?)
- Identify the WHY (is there value due to the use of technology in the course?)
- Identify the PURPOSE and METHODS OF ASSESSMENT

Many sport management programs are implementing the electronic portfolio (e-portfolio), which is an academic technology tool, into the curriculum to collect, analyze, and evaluate the types of learning and student growth taking place over a course, a semester, and even over a 4-year program of study. The key to organizing and systematically using the e-portfolio as an academic tool lies in the hands of sport management faculty members. Course by course, professors and students can develop pieces of work that capture and demonstrate student learning.

In the past students would collect documents and/or projects the dean or professor deemed appropriate. Typically, these documents provided evidence that the students met some stated competency of a program standard. Much of the collected work was placed in a binder or folder and stored in a dean's file cabinet only to be taken out to demonstrate that the purpose and mission of the program have been satisfactorily met. Those times are behind us, and we have dynamic academic technology tools that have transformed the way we can document student learning and growth. Instituting an e-portfolio into sport management programs of study can be an essential method of assessing student learning at various points in a student's academic career. Using an e-portfolio early in a sport management student's academic career creates partnerships between professor and student and student with advisor. Students have a stake and ownership in the material they contribute to their portfolio throughout the semester and ultimately throughout their 4 years in the sport management program. In addition, most if not all of the course assignments, projects, and activities are generated, communicated, and created using this portfolio model or software. The intent is to have all student-generated work in one place for easy access, easy grading, and easy reflection.

The process of instituting e-portfolio in a curriculum is time consuming and difficult when single administrators or professors go at it alone. In the end, through action research, a sport management educator can conduct pre- and post-surveys relating to the use of e-portfolios. Typically, students benefit tremendously from its use from an educational perspective, in which sport management educators can capture, collect, and analyze evidence of student growth and learning throughout a 15-week semester or term.

Getting Started: From a Professor's Perspective

A number of web-based tools can assist in portfolio creation and development. Many institutions using e-portfolio software link the data and information to the college-wide registrar or grading system to allow greater sharing of files. This relationship makes sense when we are sorting class rosters and analyzing student grades. Each sport management program should spend time researching all available e-portfolio options available in higher education. Many sport management program directors may find assistance with other on-campus programs of studies that have used e-portfolio software for a number of years for external accreditation. Creating an alliance with other departments starting to use the e-portfolio or those that are established users of the e-portfolio is a great launch for sport management programs. Some e-portfolio software allows administrators to share files across programs, which assists with rubric use and collection of students' work.

Getting Started: From a Student's Perspective

As we create a structure in sport management programs to collect and assess student learning, we must never lose focus that the intent of the tool is to foster the academic growth of out students. Students, and professors, do need to have information regarding the use and implementation of e-portfolios in their program of study. Students need to be educated on the what, where, when, why, and how of e-portfolios along with the benefits associated with its use.

Student Needs

Students need as much information as possible as to how to use the e-portfolio system. Sport management educators use e-portfolio software differently throughout the program of study, and this element must be communicated to students. Some professors may elect to promote professionally oriented e-portfolio contents for the use of practical projects, internships, and career exploration. Sport management educators may need to devote a great deal of class time to the basic elements of using e-portfolios unless another method exists. Other viable options include e-portfolio orientation outside of class or a variety of e-portfolio workshops early in the semester to assist with the starting uses of the tool. For those institutions that do not have the opportunity to meet with the entire sport management class in one designated time and place, professors must teach students, course by course, how to use the e-portfolio program.

Troubleshooting

Typically, students are either extremely excited to use e-portfolios or nervous about using this academic technology. The role of the instructor is to provide step-by-step details regarding the most simplistic elements of using e-portfolio software. Students may first need to be directed on how to purchase the software, how to log onto the software, and how to import any course-specific items (table of contents, course materials). Sport management educators who are working with first-time users of e-portfolios may need to devote either class time or office hours assisting students in the process. Once students are onboard with the basic elements of e-portfolios, sport management educators should allow students to complete work on a regular basis so that students become technology savvy and more comfortable using the new system.

e-Portfolio: Course Material

Sport management faculty members beginning the e-portfolio journey must spend time determining what methods of assessment they will be creating and collecting over the course of a semester. The opportunity to incorporate e-portfolio within the course structure can create some challenges for sport management faculty. To ease the stress, sport management departments can spend time informing and teaching each instructor about the importance of incorporating e-portfolio into the curriculum along with providing support and guidance in the transitional period. Department meetings can be filled with open discussions regarding e-portfolio from a course-specific standpoint and then as a program-wide initiative. Sport management administrators and faculty, along with reviewing the COSMA guidelines, must determine which materials will be included in student portfolios. Once course materials are highlighted for inclusion in the student portfolio, sport management faculty members can tailor the course activities and teaching methodology to meet the assessment goals of both course(s) and the overall program.

Starting the e-Portfolio Process

One of the first activities that students enjoy working on is to define and determine what a portfolio means to their academic and professional careers in sport management. Students can begin by researching definitions and descriptions of portfolios and e-portfolios. Students can determine the link between the course activities as it relates to their learning and growth with the academic discipline of sport management. Once students get a sense of the importance and role of e-portfolio in the curriculum, they will have a greater sense of ownership in the process and a greater sense of accomplishment at the end of the course.

Sample Contents for e-Portfolios: Introductory Sport Management Course

The following list can assist sport management educators in developing e-portfolio contents:

- *Defining sport management:* Students can respond, in their own words, to what constitutes sport management for their area of interest. From this starting point, students can then as a follow-up activity connect the definition of sport management (as provided through course work) to their academic and professional pursuits.

- *Sport management and you:* For this work students are asked during the first year of study to consider the courses within the sport management curriculum that are most appealing to study. The students review the list of courses within the program of study and extract goals of the course after reading a detailed course description.

- *Future courses and questions:* Students then research other class offerings at the institution they wish to complete for personal reasons and/or to supplement their professional sport management course work. Additionally, students can use this time to develop questions about specific courses they are exploring.

- *Missing courses:* At this level students can critically analyze the curriculum to ascertain if any course work is missing from the program of study. This can be a springboard to discuss the contents of material contained in some courses instead of merely reading a course title or course description that is not clear to the student.

- *Reflection:* Students, after examining the courses within the major and some from other disciplines on campus, reflect on how these courses will impact their growth and development as a sport management professional. Students indicate which professional skills they plan to develop through satisfactorily completing these courses and how these courses will support their professional ambitions.

- *Professional associations in sport management:* Students are asked to create a list of professional associations available to sport management professionals. Students are not limited in this exploratory activity. If students have a specific interest in coaching soccer they can also share their findings as it relates to those professional associations. Students summarize the mission and purpose of the association and then provide information regarding upcoming seminars or convention information.

- *Semester assignments:* Throughout the semester sport management professors can designate projects or material to be included for assessment within the e-portfolio. There are two ways to look at portfolio materials. At the course level professors should be free to create and organize the types of collected works specific to their course. For the program-wide portfolio students provide specific assignments from course work to insert for assessment within their e-portfolio. Examples of these types of activities have been explained in previous chapters of the text and can be included in student assessment portfolios and course specific portfolios.

- *Culminating project:* The final portfolio piece is an enriching exercise for students to take time to determine who they are as a person, as a college student, and as a future sport management executive. All work collected through the portfolio model from assigned course activities is now at their fingertips. The students have a chance to manipulate the collected documents and present a portfolio that gives a clearer picture of whom they are and whom they wish to become in the industry. One great learning piece of the portfolio initiative is that students have the opportunity to present their work to the class.

Teaching Tip

For online classes students have a chance to review the contents during a designated time period and post comments and questions in a forum or discussion board.

e-Portfolio Presentation

The following is an example of the final presentation of the e-portfolio material collected for an introductory sport management course. Please note, throughout the semester, a number of assessments specific to the course have been recorded for students. For the culminating project in this course, students have the chance to synthesize all their completed material, analyze the contents of the material, reflect on their growth in sport management (based on the completion of designated course activities), and finally present and demonstrate their learning and acquisition of knowledge through e-portfolio development.

Culmination of Work

Students are prompted to address content areas that can be designated by professor or program. The organization and presentation of student work can be individually crafted and designed by each student. The criteria for assessment can be manipulated by the instructor. Some examples for the evaluation criteria may include writing mechanics, reflection details and examples, demonstration of clarity in skill development, layout of portfolio, selection of artifacts, accuracy of written material and communication, and demonstration of growth and learning through reflective writing. Students must reflect on the following content areas and are also given the option to add to this list.

Introductory Sport Management Course e-Portfolio Contents

Page 1: Professional introduction, skills, aspirations, goals, and knowledge. For this section students devote time reflecting on their communicated goals listed early in the semester. From that list students now add to their goals, refine or change their goals, or enhance their goals based on the knowledge they have gained over the course of a semester and/or through practical learning activities. Students are prompted to list, describe, and reflect on five major concepts that have transformed or enhanced their vision of sport management based on course activities. Students are asked to be creative in this section to uniquely express their personal and professional aspiration in sport management and beyond.

Page 2: Internship reflection and information. For this particular course students have completed the Internship Discovery Activity (see Chapter 2). Because, at this stage, the semester is near its close, students have the collected data and information to share their journey and insight with their classmates. Often, students devote a large amount of effort in this section because internships are a major focus of achievement and stress for sport management students. Students review all research and information collected about the internship opportunities in their area of interest in sport management.

Page 3: Article reflection and insight. In this section students have a chance to extract the most important information they have gained through the collection of research on three areas of interest under the sport management umbrella. Students are prompted to communicate which articles they selected and why and extract out significant statements, passages, and quotes. Finally, students are required to share what they learned/gained from the readings. Please note, over the course of the semester, for this particular course, students collected 8 to 10 articles for review and synthesis (at varied intervals during the semester) as the information applied to them as future sport management professionals.

Page 4: Personal reflection: sport management in class discussions and information. Students were asked the following questions in the first week of the semester: why they selected sport management as a major, who they are today in the industry, and where will they be in 5, 10, and 15 years? The original statements and question responses are included in this page accompanied by new statements with highlighted changes or enhancements based on the reflected growth occurring over the last 15 weeks. The new statements must also include each student's area(s) of interest for research, practical and internship experiences in field, and career aspirations.

Page 5: Textbook reflection: chapters and learning. From the course and text readings students discuss four components that have contributed to their knowledge and insight in the major of sport management. Students select four chapters to review and synthesize the importance of the chapter information as it relates to them as future sport managers.

Page 6: A semester in review. Students are asked to share their first moments of college and class, what they were expecting, and how their vision of college and the major has changed over the course of the semester. Finally, students are asked what they are looking forward to accomplishing in the next 3 years.

Developing student portfolios is not an easy task. A culture of collaboration among sport management educators needs to be fostered and cultivated to effectively promote and use student portfolio development. Sport management programs that highlight or designate student work collected from each sport management course or from courses that address core content areas may be in a better position to pursue COSMA accreditation status than those that do not. However, we cannot assume that all professors will use e-portfolios or desire to collect portfolio artifacts in their specific courses. To resolve these issues sport management departments must create a template for all sport management instructors teaching in the program. The template provides direction for advisees and ensures the faculty members understand the role of each sport management course, including internship as we progress toward accreditation. Many sport management departments have been documenting student growth and mastery of professional competencies over the years. However, formalizing this process creates structure, uniformity, and crispness to the delivery of the undergraduate program of study. **Table 8.4** outlines the documents to be included in a student portfolio over a 4-year curriculum. The documents

Table 8.4 Sample Content for Department-Wide Sport Management Portfolio Development

---

- *COSMA principles:* Students can create a concept map connecting the courses they completed and how they have satisfactorily met the published standards.
- *Sport management coursework* (checklist of completed course): Students can review the program course of study to highlight completed courses in the major, electives, and or minors.
- *Professional information:* Students can include a resume, letters of reference, cover letter, listing of potential internship sites, and internship evaluation.
- *e-Portfolio review:* Students share and link their past work with e-portfolios created at the end of first year, second year, third year, and fourth year in the program.

Programs can decide which designated material from courses should be contained in the final program portfolio for assessment. Some examples include ethics paper (sport sociology), governance paper, sport marketing plan, policy and procedure manual, thesis paper, capstone project, and position papers.

---

can be attached to a specific course or internship experience. Attaching the work to a course makes the collection process easier because a grade (or evaluative method) may also be attached to the work.

Learner-Centered Teaching

Even with the implementation and usage of academic technology within the curriculum, we still need the human component when we are teaching and implementing a department-wide assessment system. Effective educators must still listen, respond, and continue to probe students in and out of the classroom when instituting e-portfolios.

Tools of the Industry

When we evaluate the types of technology tools our students will be responsible for using for course projects and assignments, we want to be sure there is a match with the tools most used in the daily operations of sport business. **Figure 8.1** illustrates the types of technology tools that are

Figure 8.1 Tools of the Industry

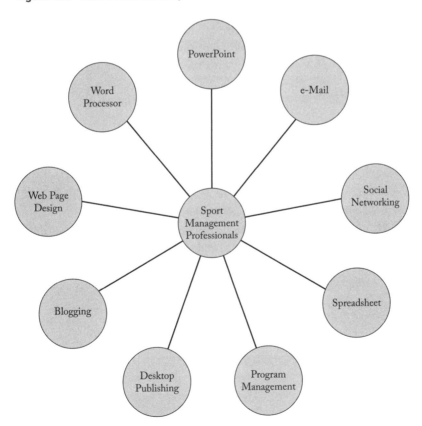

embedded into course activities and that are most likely to be used in a variety of professionally oriented sport management positions.

Questions to Consider

- Previous chapters contain a variety of activities coupled with technology integration ideas for sport management–specific courses. Technology tools can be embraced by students and enhance their level of engagement in learning. Newman (1992) defines engagement in terms of a student's level of "psychological investment" in the learning process. A follow-up question sport management professors can entertain is to determine how we (sport management) through technology make the learner feel connected or feel a strong sense of participation in the learning process?

- What technology resources and tools are you currently using in your course offerings that can be shared with other professors to collaborate and enhance the delivery of the overall sport management curriculum?

- What obstacles and challenges currently exist at your institution regarding academic technology, and what plan is in place to change the culture and provide academic technology tools to support your needs along with the needs of the program?

References

Bates, A. W., & Poole, G. (2003). *Effective teaching with technology in higher education: Foundations for success.* San Francisco: Jossey-Bass.

Gilbert, L., & Moore, D. R. (1998). Building interactivity into web courses: Tools for social and instructional interaction. *Educational Technology, 38*(3), 29–35.

Kingore, B. (1993). *Portfolios: Enriching and assessing all students* (1st ed.). Des Moines, IA: Leadership Publishers Inc.

Newman, F. (1992). *Student engagement and achievement in American secondary schools.* New York: Teachers College Press.

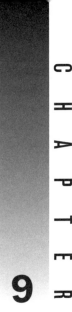

9

Outcomes Assessment

Outcomes assessment has been the academic buzz phrase for decades and will continue to be so in the future of higher education. Simply stated, outcomes assessment is investigating how well students are learning and how effectively professors are teaching students. Outcomes assessment provides the stakeholders in sport management education with an opportunity to systematically review the effects of teaching on the growth and learning of sport management students.

Organizing the process of outcomes assessment entails the involvement of both full-time and part-time sport management instructors, internship site supervisors, academic administrators, and the institution as a whole. The interconnectedness of all groups, which impacts the delivery of the sport management curricula, needs to be well grounded and organized before developing an effective and useful outcomes assessment system.

The content in this chapter includes:
- Assessment defined and explored
- Outcomes for the sport management major
- Assessment tools for sport management education

Assessment Defined

Before discussions begin on how we can determine the effectiveness of our teaching, coupled with student learning, we must create a starting point by defining assessment:

> Assessment is an ongoing process aimed at understanding and improving student learning. It involves making our expectations explicit and public; setting appropriate criteria and high standards for learning quality; systematically gathering, analyzing, and interpreting evidence to determine how well performance matches those expectations and standards; and using the resulting information to document, explain, and improve performance. (Angelo, 1995, p. 7)

Assessment provides rich data to sport management faculty members and students with information and insight to improve teaching effectiveness and learning quality. Outcomes assessment is very much action research, as faculty members have the ability to study their delivery of course content during and after each semester to improve teaching effectiveness. Outcomes assessment encourages faculty to spend time reflecting on course materials such as readings, assignments, and resources to revise or "tweak" a course to provide more effective learning outcomes. Redesigning some aspects of faculty members' courses is time consuming; however, the benefit to student learning is worth that commitment.

Program Goals and Mission

Ultimately, sport management departments need to determine and clearly state the goals for their program of study. The purpose for a goal statement or mission statement is multiple. First, sport management faculty members have the opportunity to decide the ultimate direction for the sport management department. The goals indicate to faculty members the aim for the program of study. Taking goal creation further, sport management administrators may also list a set of goals connected to each course offered for sport management students within in the curriculum. Goals ensure that faculty members (full or adjunct) understand the expectation(s) for sport management courses and for the program as a whole. As **Figure 9.1** depicts, goals can serve to connect the faculty members, connect the courses, and provide a systematic and cohesive program to sport management students.

Moving forward in outcomes assessment, we can then extract objectives from the broader goal statements. In this stage faculty members

Figure 9.1 Faculty Guidance and Input

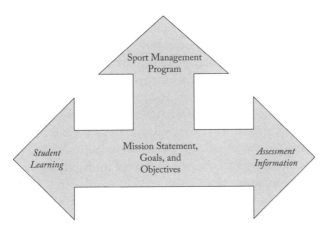

determine where their courses and course objectives "fit" into satisfying sport management program goal or goals. Goals ultimately state what the program and those who deliver the program aim to achieve. Goals are synonymous with the result; therefore the focus is not on the process or journey of learning from course to course but rather on the final product. Objectives, unlike goals, are associated with the element we want our sport management students to learn. Sport management educators use formative learning assessment throughout the course or semester. Under the formative type, assessing students occurs during the course with student participation and involvement. As indicated by Suskie (2004), "formative assessments are those undertaken while student learning is taking place" (p. 95).

The process or journey is at the heart of outcomes assessment when we consider that students are collecting knowledge as they progress from course to course, adding to their personal and professional growth that in the end typically signifies graduation. This process or journey is where teaching and learning occurs. When we consider the smaller pieces of the grand puzzle, the focus is centered on the methods in which sport management educators teach and analyze if and how much students are learning due to that teaching. On the other hand, summative assessments are final scores or grades students receive at the end of a term or semester (Suskie, 2004). Outcomes do need to provide the institution and academic administrators with what sport management students have learned and at what level of competency or proficiency as defined by the program of study. As strides are continually made in the academic discipline of sport management, so too will the methods we use to evaluate our students' growth and learning in the classroom and through integrative and internship experiences.

Outcomes for the Sport Management Major

The sport management major from a student's perspective consists of a number of courses that need to be satisfactorily completed in a designated sequence. Once the courses are complete and the grades become part of the official transcripts, students graduate with a degree. For sport management academic administrators the sport management curriculum is a listing of courses, and behind each course title contains a number of assessment opportunities to ascertain what our students are learning from our teaching and at what level of competency. To measure the skill development of students, sport management programs can create a listing of learning outcomes, which are the pathways to determine student progression and success in the program.

Outcomes assessment in sport management does not mean we exclude all learning and skill development that occurs through general education courses. In essence, sport management courses supplement the basic thinking, writing, and communication skills that are grounded within the core courses of our institutions. An example of outcomes from an undergraduate sport management major is a combination of critical thinking skills, communication skills (verbal and written), and sport management–specific content knowledge. Students may acquire these skills from courses outside of the major through satisfying college-wide core curriculum courses and from major sport management coursework as well. Sport management program directors can create a template listing of student learning outcomes, including in which courses those outcomes are addressed and evaluated.

Student Learning Outcomes

A student learning outcome, as described by Suskie (2004), is "the knowledge, skills, attitudes, and habits of mind that students take with them from a learning experience" (p. 75). As an example, an outcome requires students to explain management and apply the basic concepts of planning, organizing, implementing, and controlling to sport business. This outcome can be assessed in multiple courses, such as Introduction to Sport Management at a basic level of comprehension during the first year of the program and then again in Leadership in Sport Organizations in the third or fourth year of the program. Student work in these areas is assessed at two levels of the program, and the data can be used to evaluate the growth of the student within the major.

Most sport management programs list general student outcomes, for example, "students will be able to think critically," and specific outcomes, for example, "students will be able to compare and contrast various management theories in a logical fashion."

Assessment Tip

When creating an outcomes assessment plan, academic administrators can start by looking at the stated course objectives. Then academic administrators can meet with individual sport management faculty members to address the assessment techniques used to measure these objectives. The entire sport management faculty can then decide which courses are designated to demonstrate student learning for the outcomes assessment plan, as described in **Figure 9.2**.

There is a breadth of literature in outcomes assessment in the realm of general education and many other professional arts disciplines. Sport management educators can take advantage of the variety of methodology evaluation and assessment tools available to instructors in higher education today. The process of outcomes assessment, however, cannot be done in solitude or in a vacuum. Those institutions that provide and advocate for open discussion on assessment tools in departmental meetings are in better standing and can advance further than those that do not. Certainly, the discussion of outcomes assessment is complex, and many faculty members already believe they are actively conducting outcomes assessment through the examinations and projects they incorporate in the classroom. Other faculty members may also feel forced into adapting their teachings for the collection of student data for the purposes of outcomes assessment. Outcomes assessment planning is certainly a process whereby there needs to be a level of "buy in" from faculty members at the department level where the sport management curriculum is housed. Outcomes assessment takes time, patience, and collaborative spirit. The more sport management educators find a way to connect and learn with one another and others

Figure 9.2 Collaboration for Assessment Planning

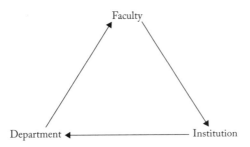

on campus that have experience in this area, the better able sport management departments are to create a cohesive academic team.

Assessment Tools for Sport Management

Over the years most faculty members have used a number of evaluative methods in their courses. There are certainly many methods included in our assessment toolbox. A list of assessment methods include written papers, tests or examinations, online discussion boards, presentations, visual performances, observation reports, interviews and analysis, quizzes, and research papers. The meaning behind these activities is what drives the assessment process. The purpose for selecting and implementing forms of evaluation must be clear and specifically related to the goals of the course and ultimately the direction of the curriculum.

Typically, we teach, we discuss, and we determine if we need to spend more time on a topic or move forward with the next series of activities. An important question is to determine what we do with the grades and work collected from an activity or after the completion of an examination. Do we make adjustments to our class lectures? Do we provide additional learning tools to be sure students understand the concepts? Do we reexamine the assessment questions to be sure we are asking the correct questions in the correct formats? Questioning our own teaching allows students and faculty in general to have an enriching educational experience with a true focus and purpose combined with identifiable outcomes.

Assessment planning promotes a program review of the assessments used for course evaluations. **Table 9.1** contains Suskie's (2004) descriptors for assessment planning using six categories: standards based, benchmarking, best practices, value added, longitudinal, and capability.

As we grade and evaluate student performance in course assignments and activities, it is essential that we determine what exactly those grades mean in regards to student learning. Angelo (1995) described a four-step

Table 9.1 Assessment Planning

---

1. Standards based: Are students meeting the standard?
2. Benchmarking: How do our students compare with peers?
3. Best practice: How do students compare with best of peers?
4. Value added: Are our students improving?
5. Longitudinal: Is our program improving?
6. Capability: Are our students doing as well as they can?

From: Suskie, L. (2004). *Assessing student learning: A common sense guide* (p. 107). Bolton, MA: Anker Publishing Company.

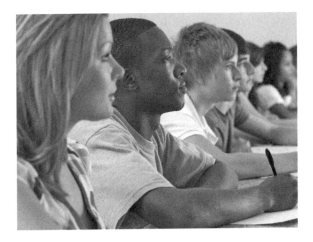

assessment cycle that can be applied to sport management that starts with defining learning goals or outcomes, then providing a variety of learning opportunities for students, then determining how to assess student learning, and finally determining to what criteria are we measuring and comparing the outcomes of student learning.

Assessment Tip

To build a collaborative effort from administrators to instructors, programs must create ways to encourage faculty development in the area of assessment. Faculty members benefit from learning about the various teaching methods that can be integrated into courses and new ways to more effectively teach students for effective learning to occur.

To develop collaboration in the assessment process:

- Conduct a workshop using an outside speaker to enlighten the faculty as to the purpose, process, and benefits of outcomes assessment.
- Provide training in methods and tools that can be easily and effectively incorporated in the classroom for the purpose of outcomes assessment.
- The process of outcomes assessment should be integrated into the sport management courses as seamlessly as possible.
- Each course should indicate learning outcomes that can be defined as what students are expected to learn after completing the course.
- Learning outcomes can also be attached to what students learn after completing the 4-year program of study.
- Faculty members and administrators need to share the information in the collection and analysis of student work.

Often, faculty members and administrators avoid at all costs voluntary participation on college-wide assessment committees. The volume of reading materials to collect and synthesis for committee-wide preparation can be a daunting task for many. However, the rewards of an organized assessment plan remain with a program for decades to follow. Embracing the concept or idea of outcomes for many in academia causes panic, and getting participation to collaborate on a committee is no easy task.

As sport management education begins to enter its adolescence in terms of an academic major, we can learn lessons of outcomes assessments from other majors on campus that have embraced outcomes assessment over the years. Nursing, education, and athletic training have been active in outcomes assessment because their external accrediting body requires documentation of learning outcomes for approval. Being able to understand and explore how those academic bodies connect all the assessment dots from course to course and for student to student to make their programs flow can be enlightening for sport management academicians.

Outcomes assessment is an ongoing process of understanding and ultimately improving student learning. The questions from students asking how they can earn a 4.0 grade point average in a class will always be ever present in higher education. The focus for faculty members committed to learning assessment should be on each of the embedded course activities that assist students in learning more about sport management and about themselves as future professionals in the industry. The purpose of assessment is to first and foremost improve student learning. Teaching effectiveness must never be ignored in outcomes assessment; conversely, the focus should remain on enhancing methods of instruction and instructional techniques.

Student Evaluations and Course Objectives: Informal Process of Evaluation

For the purposes of this section, the discussion is centered on the informal methods of class evaluations. The formal structure of student evaluations differs from institution to institution. In most cases faculty members do not have control over the questions or survey instruments being used in the formal evaluation process. In addition, the evaluation process is sensitive in nature in that student evaluations at most institutions may be tied to rank or promotion. For faculty members to learn more about their teaching methods, delivery of course content, and assessment and evaluation methods, informal student evaluations can be distributed to students, collected by the faculty member, and analyzed by the faculty member.

Assessment Tip

Ask students the questions you want them to answer. Figure out as the educator of a course what you truly want to learn from student responses. Configure your own evaluation with the statements that taps into what you want to learn from the students. Three are primary areas of exploration:
- Are the students learning through effective instruction and overall organization of the course?
- Am I using effective instruction tools to engage and ultimately teach students?
- Do the students believe they learned the important concepts of the course as outlined in the course syllabus?

Table 9.2 provides an example of an informal evaluation survey that can be used at the mid-point or end of the semester. Professors can decide whether or not to attach a grade to the assignment or not. To get a better response rate it is important to give students enough time to complete the evaluation tool. Table 9.2 is a sample evaluation tool that can be incorporated into a variety of sport management courses.

Sport Management Faculty United

The spectrum of sport management faculty members varies from those who teach sport business principles to those who focus on the sociological

Table 9.2 Final Thoughts: Sport Finance/Economics

1. Please indicate what you have learned/gained from your participation in the course.
2. What information are you unclear about?
3. List favorite elements/activities of course.
4. What were the best and worst discussion topic and chapter reading of the course and why?
5. What would you change about the course and why?
6. For an online course, did you enjoy the online format? Please explain.
7. Which topics will you continue to explore due to the course activities?
8. Please summarize (two-paragraph minimum) in your own words and using the knowledge gained from the course to respond to the following: At the beginning of the course we pondered the question is sport a big business? Now, can you describe the relationship between sport, finance, and economics? What are the key features that sustain sports into the future based on the work generated through the class?

aspects of sport. To unite the diverse group of faculty members and to be sure they all have access to the academic plan of the institution and department, several meetings should focus solely on assessment. Planning several departmental meetings to review academic offerings by semester or by academic year fosters unity among faculty members and also puts the pieces (syllabus) of the puzzle (curriculum) all together. Instructors can use this time to get feedback from colleagues, whereas new or adjunct instructors have the opportunity to determine where their course fits into the program of study. Academic administrators can use this time to connect the dots for instructors and essentially see the "big picture." This type of sharing also gets the faculty members to become a team and to realize all of the "good stuff " that they are doing within the sport management major. Most faculty members do not have time during the semester or in the hallways to share the new and innovative activities and tools they are using in their course and within their course content. Through standing and formal meetings faculty members can collaborate and assist others in adapting and improving their courses through these open sharing discussions.

In a perfect academic world we would all have an open discussion about the types of activities, projects, and assignments we use throughout the course. One way the entire program of study can be fully and effectively interconnected and tied closely together is when the department uses a portfolio system of assessment. This collection of material can demonstrate a student's growth and acquisition of knowledge in a particular area of concentration. From a micro perspective, each faculty member teaching his or her course requires students to provide evidence of mastering, reflecting, and completing activities that can benchmark a student's productivity in the class.

Using a portfolio is an effective way to determine what we are teaching and the standard(s) we use to judge/evaluate student work. The standards for projects and assignments can be connected to a rubric, which is an effective and efficient method of assessing students' work. When using a portfolio system we are able to take a macro view at the program. All the smaller essential pieces lie in each of the courses faculty members teach. The issue is to select the activities and designate the standard that is being met through the students' academic work. The process of implementing the electronic portfolio system is extremely tedious. Those involved in setting up the course content, developing standards, and attaching rubrics to student work must have a vision and be blessed with patience. Having a keen awareness of all the courses that comprise the sport management curriculum is essential. The Commission on Sport Management Accreditation principles are now the standards used to ensure students complete and achieve those established core competencies. Sport management professors also have the capability to add their own teaching touch to the portfolio that their students are using. Surely, over the next few years we will see an explosion of information relating the use of electronic portfolios within the sport management discipline.

Questions to Consider

As sport management educators and administrators proceed through outcomes assessment planning and the analysis of student progress, the following questions adapted from Suskie (2004, pp.51–52) may assist in the journey:

- Are sport management students learning what we believe is important in sport management?
- Are sport management students learning what they need to be successful as professionals in the industry?
- Should sport management educators and academic administrators modify program learning goals? Are the sport management department expectations realistic?
- Are sport management faculty members getting better at helping students learn?
- Do the assessments used give the sport management department enough information to determine students' strengths and weaknesses?

R e f e r e n c e s

Angelo, T. A. (1995) Reassessing (and defining) assessment. *AAHE Bulletin, 48*(2), 7–9.

Suskie, L. (2004). *Assessing student learning: A common sense guide.* Bolton, MA: Anker Publishing Company.

CHAPTER

10

Putting It All Together

The previous chapters covered teaching and organizational aspects of the delivery of sport management programs. Putting all the essential pieces of the sport management puzzle together presents its challenges and provides direction for students, faculty members, and administrators. Having a plan for the delivery and execution of a successful sport management program is the first step. Creating an environment in which faculty members and administrators are encouraged to share ideas and learn from one another fosters creativity and growth within the academic major. Support systems for new and established faculty members allow the groups to embrace change and celebrate new teaching methodologies and assessment techniques and tools.

This chapter covers a checklist of content that can be used to organize upcoming semesters of teaching:
- Course syllabus development
- Creation of course content (lectures, online activities, in-class exercises, exams, papers, assignments)

- Organizing assignment due dates and lecture material
- Advising responsibilities
- Mentoring students

Course Syllabus: Where to Start?

Over the years many new faculty members have contacted me asking for advice and guidance regarding the development of courses they are scheduled to teach. The process of systematically planning a 15-week, 11-week, or even 8-week course can be daunting for many whom are new to the world of teaching in higher education. One key to a successful sport management program is the relationships created and cultivated between the administrators (program director, academic dean) and its faculty members (full time, adjunct, and part time).

1. Sport management instructors can first start by asking to review previous copies of course syllabi for the course. Many program directors keep electronic or hard versions of syllabi from past years for a number of reasons, including assessment, accreditation, and internal review and/or approval.

2. For those instructors who may not have access to program syllabi, the process of course development will take more time and effort. Most institutions in higher education have approved course titles, course descriptions, and course objectives for courses listed within the college catalogs. In addition, most institutions have at the minimum a skeleton of a course that needed to be provided for institutional approval. The process of approving new courses differs from institution to institution. All faculty members should request as much information as possible regarding course syllabi before starting from scratch.

3. Professors should inquire about the various assessment tools used within the sport management program. Perhaps the sport management program is using a version of the electronic portfolio you can incorporate into the assessment and teaching activities selected for your course. Some sport management programs may require that designated examinations and/or activities are part of one course over another.

4. Course objectives are typically approved at the department level and are used from semester to semester. If there is any area missing, discuss the objective with the academic administrator for direction.

5. The course outline section of the syllabus details the daily or weekly plans for the course. Students use this section of the syllabus as a reference when planning for the assignments, projects, or examinations. Sport management educators should devote a large amount of time constructing this piece of the syllabus. Students rely on this information as they organize and balance the materials with the other courses they are completing or any outside responsibilities like sports or work.

6. Each syllabus should include a section regarding the type of assessment or evaluation of student performance that will occur over the semester or term. Students spend a great amount of time reviewing the expectations and requirements of the course to measure the amount of time and work required to satisfactorily complete the course.

7. After the evaluation section of the course syllabus, many instructors insert descriptions of each assignment listed under the evaluation section. In this area sport management students can get a deeper sense of the requirements for the course and a better understanding of the goals for each of the listed evaluation assignments.

8. Sport management instructors should also spend time customizing their course syllabus to include components that are individually important and relevant to their teaching. Some instructors include detailed information regarding late arrivals to the class (for online courses you may include logging on to the course over a 3- or 4-day period over a week), eating and/or drinking in class, plagiarism, citation of materials, class participation requirements, make-up policy, and office hour meetings.

Teaching Tip

Online courses may include log-in requirements, course participation and engagement requirements, plagiarism, citation requirements, and discussion board rubrics.

Course Content

Once the course outline is set, either by using the chapter listings from the required textbook or through the design of the instructor, sport management educators can design course notes, lecture materials, and assignments. Today, many professors use online course management systems to post all the material to be used throughout the semester. Students could use those materials as supplements to the lectures and discussions taking place in traditional face-to-face classrooms. For first-time course instructors it is important to consider the pace at which you will conduct your lectures and the timing of assignments and examinations. Please allow for changes to be made to the syllabus.

Teaching Tip

Sport management professors can use a variety of online tools, such as posting lecture slides, audio notes, and written notes in the discussion board or forum sections of the course, where the information is open for viewing and response by the entire class. With this method teaching and then learning can occur in two places: in the traditional classroom and online. Sport management professors can post or link lecture notes on the topic before the weekly assignments and then also add notes to the discussion as various teaching and learning points are developed through the online course dialogue. At the end of a teaching unit or week of activities, the sport management professor can post a summary of the discussion, tie up any loose ends on unresolved questions, and add rich information in the form of notes to assist students in come full circle of understanding the information. The sport management professor can also e-mail or post a course announcement that includes the summarized notes to the entire class to stress the importance and value of its contents. The second method of engaging the online learner is to respond directly to each of them through e-mail or designated assignment boxes. For example, if assignments are sent to the professor online or attached to a digital assignment box, professors can provide deep feedback to students in the form of a grading rubric along with narrative comments.

Teaching Tip

Many in the sport management faculty teach large courses which present challenges when trying to learn each student by name and interest in the field of study. To get a sense of each student's passion within the course, sport management educators can ask a series of questions and recorded the responses on an index card. The index card can be stored in your office and used to keep attendance or to monitor the progress of students.

Content on the index card can include:
- **Front**
  - Name
  - Cell phone number
  - Advisor
  - Sport participation on campus
- **Back**
  - Reason(s) for enrollment in the course
  - Term or semester schedule
  - Three places considering for an internship
  - Define sport management
  - List expectations of the course

Online Course Development

Clearly, all information professors provide to students in a traditional face-to-face classroom setting should be communicated to online learners. Online instructors can stress the importance of students reading and fully understanding all the elements that make up the course syllabus. Professors can create a discussion forum as it relates to specific questions regarding the course syllabus as one would if distributing the materials to a live class. Additional clarification can be provided to online students using the course website.

Course Introduction

To acquaint the online learner with your style of teaching, it is important to spend time constructing an introduction to the course. The course introduction can serve to review important concepts discussed and explored throughout the semester. Professors can also use this time to describe unique and interesting features of the course along with course objectives.

Faculty Welcome Message

All students should feel comfortable in our classrooms. Online learners appreciate an informal welcome message from the course instructor. This message can serve to develop an environment of collaboration and learning. The welcome message can be in a written posting as a course announcement or e-mail. Some instructors may consider using an audio message so that students can experience the personal touch of hearing the professor's voice. In addition, instructors can place a photo on the course website to add another dimension to the online class. At the same time students could add their own welcome message to the class. Online professors can create a welcome discussion board prompting students to post a welcome message that includes their name, nickname, reason for enrolling in the course, favorite motto or slogan, and areas of interest within the course. Students are then required and encouraged to respond to one another to learn about their interests in the course and in sport management.

Course Objectives

Course objectives are typically the same for traditional face-to-face courses and online courses. One unique feature to online course objectives is for faculty to include and highlight any unique features specific to the delivery of online materials. For instance, an objective of the course may now include the use of case study methodology that may not be used in the traditional setting.

Topical Outline

Most instructors create a detailed topical outline for the classes they instruct. For online courses the topical outline needs to be more extensive than that which is used in a traditional classroom. Instructors need to specify due dates and weekly assignments and activities to clarify the tasks for students.

Rubric for Discussion Forum Participation

Because course participation is a major component of online courses, professors must determine the quantity and quality of postings and contributions to the designated discussion boards formulated for the course. Expectations need to be set so that students are familiar with the standards and requirements of the course. To clarify the discussion forum grading, professors can create a rubric that details the specific expectations for student participation. Students should have a clear understanding regarding the expectations for the number of days per week students should participate and contribute to course discussions. Best practice in online education suggests that faculty should indicate what the standards are for superior, average, and below average responses in a discussion forum. Professors can provide examples of each category to assist the students.

Due Dates and Due Times

To ensure all of the required materials for grading are submitted to the instructor on time, it makes sense to identify specific dates and time including time zones for online courses.

Organizing Course Materials

Perhaps one of the greatest challenges for instructors teaching a course for the first time is the pace and quantity of information to be shared with students. A great resource for organizing semester-long course materials is the course schedule used by other faculty members who previously taught the course. Some professors may prepare every class lecture and activity for the term before the start of the course. Others may take into account the speed and progress of each class of students to determine the actual delivery of course material. Selecting the approach that works best for the instructor and the students is perhaps the most effective advice one can receive when preparing to teach a new course.

Advising Responsibilities

Registration Process

For many students registration for the upcoming semester can be a stressful experience. At the same time sport management faculty are also challenged by the amount of student advisees they are responsible for working with to navigate the registration process. To simplify the procedure, sport management departments can develop time-saving and useful strategies.

Sport management academic administrators should send e-mail to all sport management advisors to direct them regarding the courses students should enroll for their particular year and the designated semester. For example, first-year students who have not completed SM1XX should enroll in SM1XX before enrolling in SM2XX. The procedure can be used for student guidance at each level of study. In addition, academic administrators can prompt students to select core courses from a generated list or major courses that do not have to be completed in a sequential format. Each academic advisor can then send a personalized created message of their own to students detailing the courses they should be planning to register for in the current semester. Students need to be accountable for developing their own auditing system, and these prompts can assist in this process.

Progress Reports

Part of teaching also involves communicating grades and standard to students. Students should not be surprised when they receive a progress report. Students should be, by the time the report is submitted, keenly aware that their work and/or participation in the course needed more attention. Sport management instructors should spend time explaining the purpose of the progress report and some scenarios in which students may receive such a report. Individual professors use progress reports or the institutional academic reporting forms to encourage students to achieve at a greater level and/or seek academic assistance.

When writing a progress report, sport management professors should be as clear and concise as possible. Students should be encouraged to meet to discuss the issues with the professor before or after class or through scheduled in-office meetings if necessary.

Mentoring Students

One of the greatest joys of teaching in higher education is the opportunity to mentor students and the satisfaction of helping young professionals in sport management. The first step in the mentoring process is to be available to students.

Office Hours

Students should feel comfortable approaching professors at various times in the day. Each course syllabus should list the hours in which a professor is available for drop-in meetings (informal or formal) from students. Students in first-semester courses may also be required to schedule an appointment with each of their professors and advisor in the first weeks of the semester or term just to familiarize them with the process and to get a chance to get to know members of the academic community.

E-Mail Correspondence

Many students are comfortable sending an e-mail to address an issue or concern versus meeting a professor, in person, during scheduled office hours. Sport management professors in class and through formal advisement sessions can set the expectations of using e-mail to communicate and correspond with students. Students must understand the proper use and the etiquette of e-mail correspondence on a college campus. Often, students communicate in the same fashion as they are most comfortable with when using instant messaging or text messaging. Sport management faculty members have the opportunity, through office meetings or formal class settings, to educate students on the proper and acceptable means of communication when using technology. To create a professional correspondence with students through e-mail, professors can outline the required information. All students should include their full names in the subject along with course identifiers so the professor can have easy access to data regarding their academic records.

Value Added: Speaker Series

Inviting sport management practitioners in the industry to visit a classroom exposes students to current trends and issues within the sport business setting. Students can be required to attend on- and off-campus lectures. Sport management programs can set up a confirmation process to document the attendance and participation in these enriching academic events.

Background Information on Guest Speaker

Sport management professors can ask the invited guest speaker to provide some background information regarding their professional work that can be shared with students. The guest speaker may also provide a problem that needs to be resolved, advice or recommendations, and questions to be answered from the perspective of target markets, sport marketer, consultants, or general manager. Whether the presenter is well known, renowned, or a general contributor in the field, be sure to present the person with a token of your gratitude at the end of the session. The students should also recognize the educational presentation and the time the guest speaker devoted to traveling to the campus. Perhaps the guest speaker can follow-up with your class in future dates during the term or semester, especially if the students were charged with resolving a problem or completing an assignment.

Student Engagement During Guest Speaker Presentation

To keep students focused on the topic and the presentation given by the guest speaker, sport management faculty members must create a list of expectations:

1. Students must come prepared to the presentation with paper and pen in hand.
2. Students must research the background of the guest speaker and when available research the topic being discussed.
3. Students must create a list of 5 to 10 questions before the event they would like the guest speaker to explore during or after the presentation.
4. Students should actively take notes regarding the topic at hand and ask questions when warranted.
5. Students should prepare a written synopsis of the presentation in the form of a two-paper critique and/or review of the presentation of material.

Speaker Series Review

- List name and date of on-campus or off-campus lecture.
- Include name of speaker(s) and discussed topic.
- Describe the "lessons learned" from the speaker(s) and the overall theme of the discussion.
- Indicate your recommendation to invite these speakers to campus again or to encourage students to attend a lecture from this/these speaker(s).

Exit Interviews

Before graduation from the sport management program, academic administrators may require students to participate in an exit interview. The purpose of an exit interview is for the academic administrator to learn from the experience of the sport management students and to document the learning and growth communicated by the student due to the work within the sport management curriculum. The exit interview questions can be specific and unique to the mission of each academic sport management program with the ultimate goal to collect data to improve and enhance the quality of the educational curriculum.

Sport Management Today and Beyond

Our involvement with sport management today is dynamic and exciting. The strides and advancements of course materials and course content has evolved at a rapid pace. Opportunities for students in this energetic field of study are limitless. With new leagues and new opportunities for female athletes, more trained sport management personnel will be needed to manage and lead the industry into the next decades. Academic technology and web-based course material are changing the face of teaching in higher education. Embracing these changes will be a challenge for all of us in higher education. Moving forward into creating student-centered classrooms where the focus is on student acquisition of knowledge and the application of these core concepts in the field of sport management will be the charge for sport management programs across the globe today and into the future.

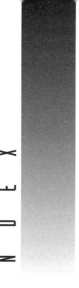

A

Accreditation
    See also Commission on Sport
        Management Accreditation
    disadvantages of, 5–6
    essential elements of field of study, 4
    statistics, 3–5
Administration. *See* Organizational
    management and administration
    activities
Angelo, T. A., 122, 126–127
Assessment
    See also Outcomes assessment
    collaboration and, 127
    defined, 122
    formative versus summative, 12, 123
    methods, 126–128
    overview of, 11–12
    planning, 126
    teaching tip, 13–14

B

Bates, A. W., 111
Boston College, 34
Branding and slogan competition, 93
Budgeting (budgets), 51–52
    creating and analysis of, 64–66
Business plan creation and analysis,
    71–72

C

Career opportunities, 55, 92–93
Charitable causes, 91
Chickering, A. W., 14
Commission on Sport Management
        Accreditation (COSMA), 5,
        114, 118
    common professional components
        (CPC), 6–8
    excellence defined by, 6
    manual (2007), 4, 6
    manual updated (2008), 4, 6
    "Outcomes Assessment Principle," 9
    standards and principles, 8,
        130–131
    technology use and, 110
Competency statements, 103
Conference affiliation activity, 40–41
Contract signing activity, 50–51
Course management systems, 22
Courses
    advising students on, 138
    content, 134–136
    grading and progress reports, 138
    objectives versus course outline, 9–10
    online, development of, 136–137
    organizing materials, 137–138
    registering for, 138
    syllabus, development of, 133–134
    teaching tips, 134, 135

D

Davis, K. A., 3

 E

Electronic portfolio
  course material, 114–116
  implementation, 111–114
  presentation, 116–119
Employment opportunities, 55, 92–93
Endorsements, professional athletes
    and, 93–94
Event creation from start to finish, 86–87
Events/contests management activity,
    51–52
Exit interview, 140–141

 F

Fielding, L. W., 5–6
Financial management activities
  budget creation and analysis, 65–66
  budget creation and decision-making
    simulation, 64
  business plan creation and analysis,
    71–72
  comparison of national versus
    international leagues, 73
  franchises/leagues, examining 70–71,
    72–73
  interview with financial manager,
    62–64
  issues for discussion, 61–62
  stock market awareness, 66–67
  stock ownership, 67–70
  teaching tips, 63, 64, 67, 68
Financial manager, interviewing a, 62–64
Foundation of sport management
  internships, 29–34
  leadership, 26–29
  resume writing, 37–38
  strategic planning, 34–37
  teaching tips, 27–29, 35–37
Franchises/leagues, examining 70–71, 72–73

 G

Games and playoffs, playing and
    scheduling, 53–54

Gamson, Z. F., 14
Gatorade, 34
Gilbert, L., 22, 111
Governance research, topics on,
    106–107
Governing bodies, 106
Guest speakers, 139–140

 H

Harvard Business Review, 97
Hiring plan activity, 55
Hybrid courses, 22–23

 I

Icebreaker activity, 26–27
International sports
  blog creation, 100
  case study analysis, 96–97
  journal presentation: global
    landscape Q & A activity, 97
  marketing activities, 97–99
  overview of, 95
  sports companies, debate issues on,
    100
  teaching tip, 100
Internet, 8
  See also Online
  web-enhanced courses, 20–22
Internships
  check-in benchmarks, 30–31
  discovery activity, 29–31
  portfolio reflection–internship
    discovery activity, 32–34
  poster presentation activity, 31
  process guide, 33
Interview
  activity, 38
  exit, 140–141
  questions activity, 37–38
  with a financial manager,
    62–64
Intramural league, creation of new, 91

 J

Jimmy Fund, 91
Journal presentation—global landscape
    Q & A activity, 97

K

Kingore, B., 111

 L

Ladies Professional Golf Association
    (LPGA), 72, 99
Laird, C., 3, 5
Leadership activities
    campus leaders, 29
    effective management and leadership,
        27
    icebreaker, 26–27
    industry leaders, 28–29
    interest group formation, 26–27
    successful managers, 28
    teaching tips, 27, 28, 29
Leagues, examining 70–71, 72–73
Learning/teaching goals/objectives
    assessment activities, 11–14
    consistency and duplication
        issues, 11
    engaging students, 14–19
    knowledge, building on prior, 10–11
    overview of, 9–10
    student summary and thoughts,
        91–92
    teaching tips, 10, 13–15, 17–19
    technology tools, integrating, 20–23
Legal aspects and activities
    case study debates, 104–105
    competency statements, 103
    debate topics, 104
    governance research, topics
        on, 106–107
    governing bodies, 106
    legal brief, composing a, 105
    overview of, 102
    professional portfolio, 103–104
    research topics, 105–106
    teaching tips, 103, 107
    topics of study, 104

M

Major League Baseball (MLB), 70, 99
Major League Soccer (MLS), 70, 72, 99
Management. *See* Financial management
    activities; Leadership activities;

Organizational management and
    administration activities
Marketing and sponsorship activities
    athletic guide, 56
    attendance, campaign to increase, 89
    branding and slogan competition, 93
    careers in sport marketing, 92–93
    charitable causes, 91
    event creation from start to finish,
        86–87
    international, 97–99
    intramural league, creation of new, 91
    mascots, changing, 88
    online discussion board, 91
    online event, interactive project, 89
    overview of, 76–77
    personalities and, 87
    products/equipment, impact of new, 88
    professional athletes and endorse-
        ments, 93–94
    promotion success or failure, 87
    publicity campaign, create a, 93
    student summary and thoughts,
        91–92
    tasks/targets, assigning, 78–86
    teaching tips, 79–80, 82, 84, 87–89
Mascots, changing, 88
Mentoring, 15, 21, 139
Miller, L. K., 5
Mission statement development activity,
    41–42
Moore, D. R., 22, 111

 N

NASCAR, 72, 89
National Association for Sport and
    Physical Education (NASPE),
    NASPE–NASSM Joint
    Committee, 4, 7
National Basketball Association (NBA),
    70, 72, 88, 99
National Collegiate Athletic Association
    (NCAA)
    compliance issues and concerns, 106
    event creation from start to finish
        activity and, 86
    job opportunities listed with, 55
    mission statement development
        activity and, 41

NCAA News, 55

NCAA.org, 55

playing the games activity and, 53, 54

schedule development activity and, 42–44, 48, 49

National Football League (NFL), 70, 72, 99

Super Bowl, 79–80, 89, 90

National Hockey League (NHL), 70, 72

Newman, F., 120

Nike, 34, 100

North American Society for Sport Management (NASSM), 3, 8

NASPE–NASSM Joint Committee, 4, 7

O

Off-season tournament development activity, 54–55

Ohio University, 4

Olympics, 89, 95

Online course development, 136–137

Online discussion board, 91

Online event, interactive project, 89

Online instruction, 22–23

See also Electronic portfolio

assessment activities, 13

debating, 100

engaging students, 15, 17

off-season tournament development, 55

principles of, 19, 22

promotions, 87

stock market awareness, 67, 68

teaching tips, 13, 15, 17

Organizational management and administration activities

athletic department flow chart, 55

budgeting, 51–52

conference affiliation, 40–41

contract signing, 50–51

events/contest management, 51–52

formation of institution, 40

games and playoffs, 53–54

hiring plan, 55

mission statement development, 41–42

off-season tournament development, 54–55

policies and procedures, 55–58

professional presentation, 58–59

schedule development, 42–49

schedule example, 43

state of athletics, 54

teaching tips, 44, 47, 48, 52, 55, 58

travel needs, 49–50

website development, 58

Outcomes assessment

See also Assessment

defined, 121, 122

faculty, uniting, 129–130

goals and mission, 122–123

for a major in sport management, 124

methods, 126–128

student evaluations and course objectives, 128–129

of students, 124–126

"Outcomes Assessment Principle" (COSMA), 9

P

Parkhouse, B. L., 4

PepsiCo, Inc., 34

Personalities, marketing and, 87

Pitts, B. G., 3, 4–5

Planning, strategic. *See* Strategic planning

Policies and procedures, activity on, 55–58

Poole, G., 111

PowerPoint, 36

Products/equipment, impact of new, 88

Professional athletes and endorsements, 93–94

Professional Golfers' Association (PGA) of America, 72, 99

Promotions. *See* Marketing and sponsorship activities

Publicity campaign, create a, 93

R

Recruiting, 56

Reebok, 100

Resume writing

feedback activity, 37

interview activity, 38

interview questions activity, 37–38

revisions activity, 37

Who am I? activity, 37

S

Schedule development activity, 42–49
Schedule example, 43
    Scheduling games and playoffs,
      53–54
Schwinn Bicycles, 34
"Seven Principles for Good Practice in
    Undergraduate Education"
    (Gamson and Chickering), 14
Slogan competition, 93
Sponsorship and marketing. *See* Marketing
    and sponsorship activities
Sport management
    accreditation and, 4–9
    defined, 2–3
    evolution of, as a field of study,
      3–4
    future for, 141
Sport Management Program Review
    Council (SMPRC), 3–4, 7
Staff policies and procedures, 56–58
State of athletics activity, 54
Stock market awareness activity,
    66–67
Stock ownership activity, 67–70
Stotlar, D., 3
Strategic planning
    benchmark assignments, 35–36
    group presentation, 36
    sport business research activity,
      34–36
    stages of, 35
    teaching tips, 35, 36, 37
Students, methods of engaging,
    14–19
Super Bowl, 79–80, 89, 90
Suskie, L., 123, 124, 126, 131
SWOT (Strengths, Weaknesses,
    Opportunities, and Threats)
    analysis, 72, 92

 T

Team building, 15–16
Technology
    See also Online instruction
    course management systems, 22
    electronic portfolio course material,
      114–116
    electronic portfolio implementation,
      111–114
    electronic portfolio presentation,
      116–119
    guide to incorporating, 20–21
    hybrid courses, 22–23
    teaching and use of, 109–111
    teaching tips, 23, 116
    types of classrooms utilizing, 22
    types of tools used, 119–120
    web-enhanced courses, 20–23
    website development, 58
Time management tips, 17
Title IX, 40, 46, 106, 107
Travel needs activity, 49–50

 U

Under Armour, 34, 67
United Way, 91

W

Web-enhanced courses, 20–23
Website development, 58
Women's National Basketball Association
    (WNBA), 70
Women's Professional Soccer (WPS), 70
World Cup of Soccer, 89, 95

Y

Yahoo.com, 67

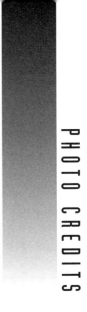

PHOTO CREDITS

Chapter 1
Page 2 © LiquidLibrary; **page 3** © Photos.com; **page 5** © Dmitriy Shironosov/Dreamstime.com; **page 12**, **page 15** © Photos.com

Chapter 2
Page 26 © Photos.com; **page 34** © David Burrows/ShutterStock, Inc.; **page 38** © Rmarmion/Dreamstime.com

Chapter 3
Page 41 © Jose Gil/ShutterStock, Inc.; **page 44** © Monkey Business Images/Dreamstime.com

Chapter 4
Page 65 © Oleg Romanciuk/Dreamstime.com; **page 66** © Lee Torrens/ Dreamstime.com

Chapter 5
Page 76 © Zairbek Mansurov/Dreamstime.com; **page 77 (top)** © Frances Roberts/Alamy Images; **page 77 (bottom)** © David R. Frazier Photolibrary, Inc./Alamy Images; **page 78** © Diademimages/Dreamstime.com; **page 80** © Ken Durden/ShutterStock, Inc.; **page 81** © Donald Linscott/ ShutterStock, Inc.; **page 83** © Rmarmion/Dreamstime.com; **page 88** © aceshot1/ShutterStock, Inc.

Chapter 6
Page 96 © Diademimages/Dreamstime.com; **page 97** © AbleStock; **page 98** © Dmitry Yashkin/Dreamstime.com; **page 101** © Alain Lacroix/ Dreamstime.com

Chapter 7
Page 105 © Junial Enterprises/ShutterStock, Inc.

Chapter 9
Page 127 © Monkey Business Images/Dreamstime.com

Unless otherwise indicated, all photographs and illustrations are under copyright of Jones and Bartlett Publishers, LLC.